POTASSIUM NUTRITION

In Heart Disease, Rheumatoid Arthritis, Gout, Diabetes, and Metabolic Shock

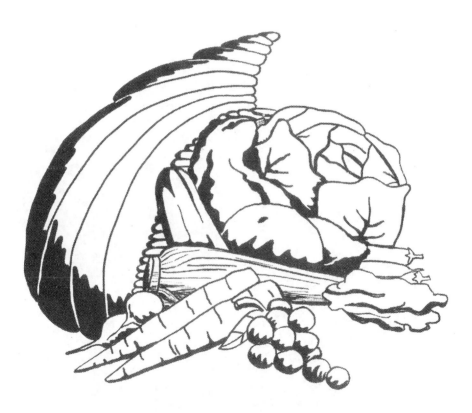

Charles E. Weber M.S.

POTASSIUM NUTRITION

In Heart Disease, Rheumatoid Arthritis, Gout, Diabetes, and Metabolic Shock

Charles Weber, MS

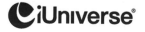

Potassium Nutrition

iUniverse books may be ordered through booksellers or by contacting:

iUniverse
1663 Liberty Drive
Bloomington, IN 47403
www.iuniverse.com
1-800-Authors (1-800-288-4677)

ISBN: 978-1-4620-1753-9 (sc)
ISBN: 978-1-4620-1754-6 (e)

Print information available on the last page.

iUniverse rev. date: 06/09/2011

TABLE OF CONTENTS

INTRODUCTION

It is my belief that a pervasive potassium deficiency caused by improper processing of food is causing a large part of the poor health in western civilization, being especially involved in heart disease, rheumatoid arthritis, gout, diabetes, and high blood pressure.

Virtually any textbook in the past would devote no more than a paragraph to potassium which would state that potassium is never deficient in the diet, or give one exception from the dozen or more known ways of loss, or in some only under clinical conditions.

The reason for this careless treatment of potassium is probably because potassium is present in almost all foods as grown in large quantities. Professionals think about it as if it were air or water. However, even air and water can be deficient and if voluminous texts are not written about those deficiencies, it is because both of those deficiencies can be detected by our senses. Extremely powerful emotions and instincts impel people to correct those deficiencies immediately and at any cost. Potassium is odorless, colorless, and, in the usual concentrations, tasteless. There is no way to detect a deficiency and cell content can not even easily be assessed in the body by modern analytical procedures other than whole body scintillation counters. Whole body cell content is virtually "invisible" other than by whole body scintillation counters.

When potassium supplements are prescribed, they get around the discordance between their convictions and practice semantically by calling the supplements "salt substitutes", "polarizing solutions", "GIK" (glucose, insulin, potassium) salts. "pharmaceutical affecters", "ORT salts (oral rehydration therapy for diarrhea)", or similar terms. A deficiency is further defined out of existence by defining the blood serum content is normal at a 4.2 Meq/liter when the actual figure is 4.8 [Scribner].

Psychic stress stimulation of aldosterone, diarrhea (Potassium supplements to babies brought mortality from a virulent strain of diarrhea from 35% to 5% [Darrow]), profuse perspiration, excessive vomiting, eating sodium carbonate or bicarbonate (because hydrogen ion is excreted at the same site as potassium), laxatives, diuretics, licorice, hyperventilating, enemas, shock from burns or injury, hostile or fearful emotions, and very high or low sodium intakes all increase potassium losses, some massively. All together would probably be lethal in a fairly short time. Reliance on grain (especially white flour) or fatty foods, boiling vegetables, use of chemicals (soft drinks, for instance) instead of food, and use of most processed foods including frozen and canned permit considerable reduction of intakes. So does the reduced appetite associated with a sedentary life.

To speak of potassium deficiency as an aberration when enormous numbers of people are affected by these circumstances and our food is so badly damaged is not logical. Even if a serious degenerative disease does not materialize, an adequate intake is desirable to forestall future disasters and to permit one to operate at optimum. Some of the manifestations of the placebo effect become understandable in light of the affect of emotions on electrolyte hormones. However, we cannot always be assured of a placebo being available, certainly not on the firing line, but not even for that matter in the quiet of a hospital where even nurses can be testy at times.

It is especially important that nutrition be established by experiment. Currently, every one in the medical establishment is convinced that potassium deficiency cannot be involved in rheumatoid arthritis, but this with only one experiment ever having been performed. It simply is not possible to predict the outcome of an experiment with certainty without actually performing it. It would be desirable to determine the affect of every food common in commerce not only on arthritis, but on all the degenerative diseases. Some foods, known to be poisonous to animals or have poisonous related species in the wild, have been used for thousands of years without ever having been tested. This is undoubtedly due to a universal quasi religious conviction or instinct that foods our parents taught us to eat or taste good could not possibly be harmful. This is not necessarily the case. Such experiments could have another advantage in that they might uncover foods that have a beneficial effect. Even small effects would be worth knowing about. The above conviction (or instinct) is so strong that most people will not eat nutritious food if tastier, but less nutritious food is available. Their instincts override their intellect not only in their eating habits, but in their scientific efforts. These scientific efforts are further thwarted from pursuing nutritional investigations because medical science stresses pharmaceuticals and glamour theories [Forman].

Please keep in mind, though, that potassium ramifies through every cell and process in the body, has almost no storage, and has a dangerous dependence on its precise control for nerve impulse transmission. This makes it a mineral to be cautious about. In particular I recommend getting as much as possible from food. Even food requires a little care because it has a wide range of concentrations. You must take responsibility for your own intake and I assume no liability for the correctness of advice in this book. You use this information at your own risk. Also please keep in mind that some of the information in this book is based on poorly performed experiments or biased commercial sites. If you have a medical problem, be sure to seek the consultation of a medical or nutritional professional. Such a person has more information available than just potassium nutrition and, perhaps equally important, is in a position to run tests.

Anything a doctor or dietitian can learn about nutrition, you can also. If you do not know the meaning of a word in these articles, for a definition click on http://www.m-w.com (Mirriam-Webster), or http://www.nlm.nih.gov/medlineplus/encyclopedia.html (a medical encyclopedia) or http://www.wikipedia.org (a comprehensive encyclopedia).

The health of people in the USA is abysmal (numerous statistics here [http://www.foodrevolution.org/roh_facts_print.htm]), and a major part of it is poor nutrition. Vegetable oils and refined sugars, which are essentially devoid of potassium, make up one third of the total food energy. Displacement of vegetables and fruit by whole grains and milk products further reduces the potassium intake because potassium concentrations in vegetables are four times and twelve times those in milk and whole grains, respectively, whereas in fruit the potassium concentration is two and five times that in milk and whole grains. The disaster is made much worse by refining of whole grains, which white flour has only one quarter the potassium of whole grain. Added to this is the ingestion of huge amounts of sodium chloride salt, beyond anything the body can easily handle.

As the 12th century physician, trying to cure by diet before he administers drugs, said; "No illness that can be treated by diet should be treated by any other means" or as Hippocrates expressed it in 460 - 377BC; "If we could give every individual the right amount of nourishment and exercise, not too little and not too much, we would have found the safest way to health". It would seem that a healthy life style has been known for a long time. It is my belief that an unprocessed, unfrozen, not canned, high in vegetables, free of poisons diet would keep a large majority of people reasonably healthy and without the need for fad diets. 80% of Americans do not eat adequate vegetables, but even though 72% of Americans take vitamin or mineral supplements daily or occasionally, their health is atrocious. These supplements never include significant amounts of potassium with vitamin pills. Even potassium pills have only a tiny amount. Fairly significant amounts would be obtained if a dozen or two were taken each day (see chapter 8 before taking any). Very few do so though.

I would suggest that a partial solution to the problem of poor potassium nutrition would be to place a tax on all food that has had potassium removed by food processors and completely fund all Medicare and workman's compensation for injuries and disease that relate to rheumatoid arthritis, gout, heart disease, strained ligaments, and high blood pressure. This would also take the Medicare and Medicaid onerous tax burden now incurred for them and place it on the shoulders of those who cause the problem.

All the references are gathered together at the end and organized according to chapters except URLs, which follow statements pertinent to them. You may see a site that has links to words used in nutritional and biological science in [http://lpi.oregonstate.edu/infocenter/minerals/potassium/]

I repeat, I assume no liability for statements in this book. They are sometimes based on flimsy evidence. Of course, better flimsy evidence than no evidence at all. But in any case I do not want anyone getting sick from a miss print and then even so much as becoming irritated with me.

CHAPTER 1
POTASSIUM IN FOOD

SUMMARY

This chapter describes the situation of the potassium status in food. Food is the most important part of our environment. Our health and our very life depends on food. So it is imperative to know this. So be sure to read which foods contain the most potassium, where you can find exact amounts, and how the amounts are expressed and why.

The richest sources of potassium are leafy vegetables low in starch. The reason why starch reduces the amount of potassium per calorie is that potassium does not enter the plant cell associated with starch. This is unlike animal starch, called glycogen, which has to be associated with potassium inside the cells.

All whole foods contain potassium before being processed. Starchy vegetables such as bananas and potatoes contain moderate amounts of potassium, about 4 milligrams per Calorie. Meat low in fat contain an amount that would support life under normal circumstances, about 2,5 milligrams per calorie. This amount will usually support life. The reason why fat decreases the amount of potassium per Calorie is that fat is high in Calories but contains virtually no potassium because potassium is not soluble in fats and oils.

Large amounts of potassium are possible from food alone as some South American Indians receive over 8 thousand milligrams per day from their food [Oliver]. The reason why people in western civilizations do not get enough potassium, white people in Georgia, USA, averaging 2000 milligrams per day and black people 1500 milligrams, is that almost every food processing procedure loses potassium. Also some foods are added to processed foods that have no potassium in them, such as sugars, fats, oils, and starch. The amount of potassium that will just barely maintain optimum health in the absence of infectious diseases, perspiration, or genetic defects is about 2500 milligrams per day.

When attempting to increase our potassium, it is desirable to know which foods are high in potassium. It is not sufficient to know the amount of potassium in a given weight of food. What determines how much food we eat is largely determined by the number of calories contained in the food. We eat until our appetite is sated by a sufficient intake of food energy, and then we tend to lose our appetite. Therefore information on potassium in foods is much more useful if it is expressed as weight of potassium per Calorie [Weber 1974].

I show two tables in chapter 13 and 14 that give potassium contents this way. Table 1 (chapter 13) lists foods in alphabetical order. Table 2 (chapter 14) lists foods in order of decreasing potassium.

The justification for using Calories contributed by fat or oil in the potassium in foods tables depends on the assumption that fat and oil contribute as much to appetite suppression as do carbohydrates. This is not the case short term [Blundell]. However this approach is still justified because trained muscles burn fat as well as carbohydrates [Saltin] and everyone except chronic fatigue syndrome (CFS ME, or CFIDS) victims should get as much exercise as possible for there is said to be no damage to the joints. While moderate to heavy exercise has been shown to be beneficial to fibromyalgia (probably a CFIDS variant) [Hadhazy], exercise in a pool has been shown to give improvement in pain, anxiety, depression, and number of good feeling days were more evident than land exercise [Jentoft]. I suspect that many short sessions of mild exercise across the day would be the best way, probably for rheumatoid arthritis also. Furthermore the foods which I recommend are low in fat and under such circumstances a high proportion of the fat is either burned or stored in the body's fat cells [Westertape] anyway. Therefore ultimately most of the fat and oil in a healthy diet contributes to appetite suppression long term and therefore probably no useful purpose would be obtained by attempting to compute a weighted factor against the fat contribution. A diet high in fat and oil is disadvantageous for other reasons, such as flushing out fat soluble vitamins, so no net problem should arise including fat calories.

As you can see, if potassium content is expressed as milligrams per Calorie, most foods lie between 0 and 10 milligrams per Calorie and few are higher than 20. These are convenient numbers, easy to read, and make a good comparison for foods when assessing their relative potassium contents. Such a designation is much more useful in attempting to decide which foods to eat than a "per serving" designation which gives very little hint as to relative value and a per weight basis for dry foods is actually misleading.

The Table from which these values were computed may be seen in http://www.nal.usda.gov/fnic/cgi-bin/nut_search.pl . To access the information you must press "enter" to search, and then divide Kcal into milligrams of potassium. That last table is very comprehensive, is used in search mode, and even lists all the amino acids. It is available in a PDF printable form for potassium only also in http://www.nal.usda.gov/fnic/foodcomp/Data/SR15/wtrank/sr15a306.pdf . There are also links to PDF types of printouts from the table for other individual nutrients available in http://www.ars.usda.gov/Services/docs.htm?docid=9673 . Just click on the "A" or "W" button for the nutrient that you wish. A site is available which shows foods which are high in one nutrient and low in another (including calories) in http://www.nutritiondata.com/nutrient-search.html.This last site should be especially useful for a quick list of foods to consider first, or for those people who must restrict another nutrient.

KITCHEN LOSSES OF POTASSIUM

At least one of the industrial processes is possible in the kitchen for losing potassium, and is a characteristic way of cooking vegetables in America. Whichever vegetables are boiled suffer losses equivalent to processing losses if fresh, or often can suffer further losses if they have already been processed. Unless salt is present in the boil water or canning liquids, there is a limit to how much potassium can be lost. This is probably because large negatively charged molecules can not diffuse out of the heat damaged cell wall, and the charges inside the cell must remain balanced. This limit appears to be over 50% for most vegetables. The losses tend to be greater with larger amounts of water and longer boiling times, but apparently not always. The losses are unnecessary. There are numerous ways of cooking vegetables so that there are no losses at all, and several where the losses are small. It is important to know how to cook food properly because some foods can not be eaten at all raw and many foods a cause poor growth rates when eaten raw, such as legumes, probably because interfering materials in some vegetables are destroyed by the cooking. Baked or broiled vegetables retain everything except a fairly large loss of vitamin C and lesser losses of some of the B vitamins [Pearson][Krehl]. Usually only potatoes and stuffed peppers are baked, but in theory all foods could be baked or microwaved. One way to cook food in a microwave which would lose so much moisture if baked so that they would not taste good, would be to place them in a casserole or closed pot along with a small amount of water. Meat which is broiled sometimes actually increases in potassium content if fats are rendered out of them. Pumpkins and squash can be baked right in the shell if they are punctured to avoid exploding. It is easy to make pudding after baking them. If a young pumpkin or squash is used it is possible to eat it seeds and all. I have no analysis of the seeds.

In order to gain the greater speed that using the top of the stove implies you could fry the vegetables. This is already often done with onions, potatoes, mushrooms, eggplant, peppers, squash, and tomatoes. Many vegetables which are difficult to fry can be fried by placing them in the pan with vegetables which are easy to fry. Oil is often used to prevent sticking to the pan. A small amount of oil for frying is much preferable to boiling and discarding the boil water. It is even conceivable that a small amount of unhydrogenated vegetable oil may be a nutritional plus if it is high in omega 3 oil. If a Teflon coated pan is used with careful control of heat, no oil at all needs to be used.

Actually it is not the boiling itself which is bad, but the subsequent discard of the water, If the cook were to retain the water as when making soup or for use when boiling future vegetables the situation is solved, for if they are not allowed to boil dry, there are no losses at all. The boil water can also be used as a beverage. It is especially tasty when derived from mixed vegetables (to my taste buds). This would be a way of augmenting your potassium intake if your family would be willing to grant you more than your fair share of the liquid when pulling out of a deficiency.

If small amounts of water are used in closed pots, known as steaming, the losses should be minimized. I have no analysis available for this procedure, but my knowledge of the physical chemistry involved makes me suspect that the losses are small. If the liquid at the bottom of the pot is used, there are no losses at all. Pressure cooking is a form of steam cooking. It is much faster and less likely to run dry. I do not have information of its affect on heat sensitive vitamins.

Microwaving should lose no potassium but I have no analysis.

Gravies and drippings consisting of watery material are usually rich in potassium. You should always make an effort to sop up, spoon up, or drink up the watery liquids on the bottom of your plate or in the pan while attempting to leave the fats behind. If it is impossible to separate them, it is often possible to skim the solid off the top after a sojourn in the refrigerator. Decanting fat off of a tall glass is another possibility.

TABLE SCRAPS

Another loss, although not strictly a processing loss, is the tendency to leave food on the plate when not very hungry. The foods which are most likely to be left by most people are precisely those foods which are highest in potassium, the vegetables. One way to avoid this type of loss would be to eat the most nourishing food first. So far as cooking is concerned the cook should make a considerable effort to make the vegetables appetizing. Like Popeye the sailor, concentrate on the vegetables. There are numerous combinations with milk, meat, spices, fruits, and other popular foods which can make vegetables anywhere from palatable to irresistible. Just combining several miscellaneous vegetables can be a considerable improvement in taste.

      The following table lists some food combinations which I have found to be better tasting than either alone, or at least better than the first on the list. Some of those on the left side of the list are almost intolerable alone.

FOOD COMBINATIONS

asparagus---------------------------- milk
bean seeds-------------------------- tomato
beans, green----------------------- milk
beans, lima------------------------ corn
beets ---------------------------------- milk and/or vinegar
bran---------------------------------- raisins and milk
cabbage------------------------------ buttermilk or yogurt
carrots, raw ------------------------ raisins
carrots, cooked --------------------- peas
celery --------------------------------- lettuce and apple
chives -------------------------------- cottage cheese
cress, water-------------------------- other salads
cucumbers -------------------------- vinegar or sour cream
liver ---------------------------------- onions, fried
milk---------------------------------- carob powder or chocolate
oatmeal----------------------------- apples, bananas
parsley ------------------------------- potatoes
peppers, sweet --------------------- meat
peanuts ------------------------------ dates
pumpkin, mashed---------------- eggs, milk, and cinnamon
spinach, raw ----------------------- other salads
spinach, cooked -------------------- milk
wheat germ ------------------------- meat loaf or cereal
yeast --------------------------------- milk
yogurt ------------------------------- strawberries

CHAPTER 2
OTHER NUTRIENTS

SUMMARY

Discussed here are the characteristics of each of the three main food groups, animal sourced, vegetables, and grains with fruit. Potassium and its interactions are stressed, but other nutrients are also discussed, especially if they are likely to be deficient in our society.

Take a look at a marvelous site that gives average RDR multiples for most of the essential elements in graphical form from several food groups along with average costs [http://www.vegsource.com/harris/ten_categories.htm]. Vegetables are the winners.

You may also see graphs and tables describing the changes that have taken place in our diet from our stone age ancestors by Cordain, et al, in [http://www.ajcn.org/cgi/reprint/81/2/341.pdf].

MEAT, FISH, MILK, CHEESE, AND EGGS,

We depend on these for high quality protein (especially methionine and lysine), sodium, chloride, iodide and vitamin B-12. Vitamin B12 is said to be also present in spirulina, or blue green algae, but is thought to be an analogue of B-12 [http://www.vegsoc.org/info/b12.html], which could conceivably make a deficiency worse. Fermenting vegetables will not provide adequate vitamin B-12 [Rauma 1995 with comments in 1997]. Red Star T-6635+ yeast is said to be rich in vitamin B-12 derived from bacteria. I do not know if it is a useful form. [http://www.vegansociety.com/html/food/nutrition/b12/] All vitamin B-12 comes from micro-organisms and is not normally harmful in excess. If a deficiency is relieved by supplements, the sudden surge in red cell metabolism can cause a sudden drop in plasma potassium severe enough to be life threatening [Lawson] so supplements of potassium should be used. A vitamin B-12 deficiency is very dangerous, especially in babies [http://www. hacres.com/pdf/documents/B12-Hallelujah-Diet-Donaldson.pdf].

VEGETABLES,

These we depend on for vitamin A, vitamin C, and potassium. They are also good sources of all the other vitamins and minerals except those listed under meat above, and vitamin D, which is not really a vitamin, but a hormone. To the extent that it is de facto a vitamin for those working and studying inside, it is present in liver, sardines, irradiated milk, cod liver oil (However there should not be more than 10 times as much vitamin A in any supplement since, while sufficient vitamin A is thought to be essential to vitamin D's proper functioning [http://foodconsumer.org/7777/8888/N_ utrition_35/121009342008_Don_t_use_cod_liver_oil.shtml], too much is thought to interfere with vitamin D) and tablets. It is said that a naked white man receives 20,000 IU of vitamin D within a few minutes of bright sunlight, well before tan or burn [http://www.ndmnutrition.com/vit.%20d%20inflam]. It is necessary in the body to guard against tuberculosis [Wilkinson], to gain calcium for avoiding bone loss, to possibly inhibit cancers, and to retain magnesium. It has been proposed that vitamin D has an affect dampening the immune system, especially with regard to multiple sclerosis [Cantorna]. It is more likely that the affect on magnesium is involved, and thus indirectly powers the potassium cell wall pumps, for which magnesium is required [Grace] (see chapter 3 and 8 for extensive discussion) or by powering the calcium cell wall pumps affects pain. The optimal values in the blood are proposed as 45-50 ng/ml or 115-128 nmol/liter of vitamin D. We are now better able to identify sufficient circulating 25(OH)D levels through the use of specific biomarkers that appropriately increase or decrease with changes in 25(OH) D levels; These include intact parathyroid hormone, calcium absorption, and bone mineral density[http://jn.nutrition.org/cgi/content/full/135/2/317]. Using these functional indicators, several studies have more accurately defined vitamin D deficiency as circulating levels of 25(OH)D ≤80 nmol or 32 µg/ Liter. Recent studies reveal that current dietary recommendations for adults are not sufficient to maintain circulating 25(OH)D levels at or above this level, especially in pregnancy and lactation. There has been established a wide margin of safety above current intakes [http://www.ncbi.nlm.nih.gov/ pubmed/17823429].

It has been proposed that vitamin D accentuates the symptoms of sarcoidosis (thought to be a bacterial infection) [http://sarcinfo.com/faq. htm], and supplements or sunlight probably should not be used then. Antibiotics have been used successfully against sarcoidosis [http://yarcrip. com/sarcoidosissuccumbs-preprint.htm]. Those authors believe that a mycoplasmin like bacteria is responsible for that disease, and suggest that similar bacteria may be involved in rheumatoid arthritis and other diseases like it by infecting white blood cells and causing autoimmunity. So it is also possible that the vitamin D is having a direct affect on rheumatoid arthritis if arthritis is indeed an intracellular infection (see chapter 11), for it has been discovered that vitamin D activates a cell receptor that activates antimicrobial peptide (cathelicidin), which is involved in killing of intracellular bacteria such as tuberculosis bacteria [Liu]. Apparently epidemiological studies and circumstantial evidence show lower rates of multiple sclerosis, hypertension, osteoarthritis, colorectal, prostate [Chan], inflammation, influenza, tuberculosis, breast, and ovarian cancer, [http://archinte.ama-assn.org/cgi/ content/abstract/168/11/1174] and heart disease, when vitamin D is adequate [Tavera-Mendoza]. Perhaps water companies should put vitamin D in water instead of that awful poisonous, destructive fluoride.

GRAINS AND FRUIT,

These are primarily cheap or tasty sources of calories. Grain price is made even artificially lower in the USA since 90% of subsidy payments were authorized to farmers of corn, wheat, oil seeds, rice, and cotton [Doyle]. Grains also provide a fair amount of Vitamin E and B vitamins (other than B-12). Fruits are usually fair sources of potassium and vitamin C. Foods that contain 1 milligram per Calorie or better of potassium, as do whole grains, would probably meet the minimum daily requirement for most young people. This assumes a person in good health who burns 2,500 Calories per day, which would yield the 2,500 milligrams per day or so that is probably the minimum requirement. It also assumes no drains on potassium from stress, disease (such as diarrhea), perspiration or other losses. The only time that it would be necessary to eat grains would probably be if the only vegetables eaten were leafy ones low in calories and heavy work were being performed, for it is said that celery has negative calories, for instance. That is, it takes more calories to eat a piece of celery than the celery has in it to begin with. It is said to be the same with apples. These last statements are no doubt exaggerated somewhat. Grain contains very little or no vitamin A, C, or D.

MEAT: EXTENDED DISCUSSION.

Lean meat low in fat has fairly consistent amounts of potassium, usually about 2 mg/Cal. It can range from 1 to 3 mg/Cal. Because fats or oils have no or little water to dissolve potassium, and because they are high in calories, they are very low in potassium, approaching zero. Therefore meat with much fat in it will be lower in potassium per calorie than lean meat. It is important not to eat charred part of meat since there is some evidence that chemicals there can cause cancer. Milk compares to meat as a source of potassium, and has the same dependence on fat content. The lactose in milk is difficult to digest for adults outside of the Caucasian and Semitic races and causes digestive upsets. That problem can probably be solved by adding the proper enzyme to the milk. Also, milk is very low in copper, and copper is necessary to repair cartilage damaged by both kinds of arthritis to achieve maximum strength [Weber 1984], to maintain cross linking of the elastin tissue in blood vessels, and to prevent too high a cholesterol content..

Eggs, like meat, are an excellent source of protein, and for normal people should make a good adjunct to the diet. You should bear in mind, however, if you are in the throes of recovering from a deficiency, that they are low in potassium. This would be expected, since the developing chick is trapped inside the egg. It has no way of excreting potassium and must end up with the correct amount, after burning some energy and making some feathers. Eggs have been given some bad press because of the cholesterol hypothesis. However there are tribes, which eat large amounts of eggs in Africa, that have a much lower heart disease rate than we do. The Masai tribe members have low cholesterol [Brown p8-9] even though heart disease is a problem with them. Low cholesterol diet has little affect on cholesterol [http://www.ravnskov.nu/myth3.htm] because high blood cholesterol is probably due primarily to impaired conversion of cholesterol to bile acid [Mann p647], which is probably usually caused by a copper deficiency, and an egg a day has no affect on cholesterol [Slater] [Hu], and Cholesterol lowering drugs give a higher death rate [http://www.health-heart.org/causes.htm] [Mann p646], and the cholesterol level is normal in the average heart attack victim. In fact, too little cholesterol in the body can cause health problems [http://www.ctds.info/low_cholesterol.html]. A higher cholesterol intake increases sterilization of tuberculosis bacteria by the body [Perez-Guzman], so must be desirable in immunity. High sodium chloride (table salt) intake for 1-4 years has been found to frequently cause high blood cholesterol [Dahl]. The erroneous attitude of the medical profession toward cholesterol has been ascribed to misinterpretation of the data and lack of precision in semantics [Stehbens]. Nicotinic acid (vitamin B3a) is said to have the affect of lowering the undesirable form of cholesterol [http://www.innvista.

com/health/nutrition/vitamins/b3.htm]. For some side effects of cholesterol lowering drugs see links in this site [http://www.thincs.org/unpublic.htm] Golomb and Marcella have written a review of the [http://cardiovascular. adisonline.com/pt/re/cvd/abstract.00129784-200808060-00004.htm;jsessi onid=JQ7C382VNKdSbB324BPv1Xd0sPLJyFJc6KdntPppbFCFKGDhry6 T!136317464!181195628!8091!-1] affects of statin drugs on the body and have concluded the bad side effects of those drugs are because of inhibition of mitochondrial activity.

There have been affective treatments rejected in the past solely because they did not conform to mistaken accepted hypotheses [Goodwin]. So eggs should make a reasonable source of protein for everyone. It is said that prolonged salt intake can also raise cholesterol, as mentioned above. Most of the potassium is concentrated in the white of the egg. Egg whites are comparable to meat in content, and are in fact higher than most meat. One way to make a slight gain in potassium intake, if you are the only one deficient in your family, is to have your portion of the egg high in the whites until any deficiency symptoms disappear.

It is also said to be important to receive at least a small amount of meat or dairy products at every meal for adults because these are quality proteins. Many nutritionists believe that you should eat more than the 50 grams of protein in a 2000 Calorie diet, which the US government recommends, as much as double that amount or more. I can not help with advice on this for sure, but I suspect the government's recommendation is a minimum or worse. Much of the usefulness of quality protein (protein high in lysine and methionine amino acids) is said to be lost if it is eaten even as little as two hours after the main meal..

Lysine can have some additional importance because arginine amino acid accentuates the symptoms of an attack of the herpes type of virus [McCune] (such as chicken pox, shingles, infectious mononucleosis, roseola). Thus an attack of shingles, which disease is a resurgence of chicken pox virus from the pain nerves near the spine where they have been dormant, will be accentuated and perhaps even triggered by foods high in arginine. These foods are said to include peanuts (peanuts are 50% higher than cashews, but which last are substantial nevertheless), other nuts and non grass seeds, and chocolate. See here for a table which gives lysine and arginine values by weight of food and lysine\arginine ratios [http://www.herpes.com/Nutrition.shtml]. Lysine helps to mute the effects of the virus, significantly reducing the occurrence (when taken routinely during the disease), severity, and healing time of herpes simplex virus [http://www.healthy.net/asp/templates/article. asp?PageType=article&ID=1744] [Griffith]. You can recognize shingles by large patches of a painful rash which appears on one side of the body in people under emotional stress [Irwin], older people, or people whose immune system has been compromised. There is a potassium chloride table salt on the market that contains lysine to mask the potassium flavor [http://www.alsosalt.com/nutritionfacts.html]. It may prove to be a good source.

It is said that injections of adenosine monophosphate and interferon gamma will also help heal herpes infections [Nikkels].

VEGETABLES: EXTENDED DISCUSSION

Vegetables, low in starch, are the best sources of potassium. They rarely go below 5 mg/Cal., and range up to 20 mg/Cal. or more. The seaweeds are poor sources of potassium. An additional reason I can not recommend them as a substantial replacement for vegetables, however, is because of their high salt content and because they contain bromine and arsenic (22 milligrams of arsenic per 1000 grams) in it, both largely as organic compounds. Between 0.2 to 1.0 milligrams per day of arsenic is ingested by the Japanese daily. Inorganic arsenic is a risk factor for liver cancer. However hijiki seaweed has only 0.3 milligrams per 1000 grams of arsenic as arsenate, the remainder being organic, which is only mildly toxic. The UK Food Standards Agency (FSA) issued advice to consumers to avoid eating seaweeds. Iodide is an antidote of sorts for bromide and fluoride poisoning [http://findarticles.com/p/articles/mi_m0ISW/is_2003_May/ai_100767875]. Of course the best way to avoid fluoride poison is to not drink fluoridated water, bathe in it, or eat food with fluoride insecticides on it. The Japanese average 13.8 milligrams per day iodide from seaweed [Nagata]. Stadel proposed that the low incidence of breast cancer in the Japanese (Iceland also has a low rate and high iodide intake) is due to their high iodide intake [Stadel] and this has been confirmed [Funahashi]. Selenium is synergistic with iodide for that purpose [LeMarchand] [Nagata]

If you wish to increase the variety or taste of the vegetables which you eat by growing your own perennials there are sites which lists growth parameters of trees and shrubs [http://www.efn.org/~bsharvy/edible.html]. --or-- [http://www.naturalhub.com/natural_food_guide_vegetables.htm]

That second site discusses wild vegetables which are edible, and some evolutionary aspects of vegetable eating. One thing folks can do to help with vegetables that form from flowers, even if you aren't a beekeeper, is to make your yard bee friendly. Plant a flowering herb garden. Bees use herbs medicinally and your plants can help make a difference. It has been suggested to use rosemary, sage, THYME (lots of it), marjoram, chives, basil, all the mints and other herbs with flowers. Perhaps even better, it is said that short bamboo pieces lashed together in a tree will give one of the bee species a home.

GRAIN AND SEEDS: EXTENDED DISCUSSION

Grain and seeds [http://www.naturalhub.com/natural_food_guide_grains_ beans_seeds.htm] (see evolution of seeds as food [http://www.webmd.com/a-to-z-guides/features/eat-your-vegetables-15-tips-for-veggie-haters?ecd=wnl_ din_020209&?wpisrc=newsletter]) are a major part of the World's calories Wheat alone provides 20% of the calories [Uauy]. Grains are the lowest in potassium of the major categories, and will usually run about 1 mg/Calorie of potassium. Nuts are similar to grain. The bean, peanut and legume seeds are a fairly good source, usually running about 3-4 mg/Calorie. They along with chocolate and some other nuts are high in arginine amino acid which apparently should not be eaten when suffering from a herpes viral infection such as chicken pox, shingles, genital herpes [McCune] or fever sores (see further discussion below). When first recovering from rheumatoid arthritis or other potassium deficiency and attempting to build up your body's potassium, it would be well to use whole wheat bread and cake sparingly (and no refined flour products at all, ever). Substitute wheat germ and yeast for some of it and vegetables for the rest. People who are intolerant of gluten protein should eat no wheat at all. A very important consideration is to eat extremely sparingly of foods containing large amounts of sugar, starch, or fat, regardless whether the sugar, starch, or fat was placed there naturally or by the hand of man because no potassium is associated with those substances. Refined flour is extremely low in potassium but is not part of this discussion since no one should ever be using that useless rubbish under any circumstances because of a number of other deficiencies. It is too bad that the aristocracy's adoption of white flour in days of yore got all of us peasants hooked on that junk. How it happened is a testament to our admiration for the rich and famous. It happened even though whole wheat tastes much better than that bland junk in my opinion.

A diet high in protein has been touted as superior to carbohydrates and for people who have not lost kidney function or have not cured their gout it is probably acceptable. However, the main reason why carbohydrates have received a bad perception is probably because the criminally incompetent jerks in the processed food industry have evolved clever ways to remove or destroy essential nutrients in carbohydrates, sometimes 100% of them (white sugar, for instance).

When people speak of a balanced diet, they usually mean that you should get a fair share of each category of food each day. By so doing you make it unlikely that there will be too little or too much of any essential nutrients. If you get about equal calories from each of the three categories, you should have a reasonably balanced diet as defined by the crude definition at the beginning of this paragraph and most people will be reasonably healthy. However grain and fruit are not essential. You can probably get all your nourishment from meat and vegetables, and it is undoubtedly a superior way to eat [LaVecchia et al] [Van Duyn]. I do recommend that you include wheat germ in your diet though, because it is unusually rich in vitamin E and is a very good source of omega-3 oil and the B vitamins other than B-12. In addition, there is a suspicion that some unessential compounds in vegetables can have desirable affects against other diseases. One such desirable compound in cashew nuts is anacardic acid, which is extremely lethal to the gram positive bacteria that cause most tooth infection and will cure that kind of tooth infection or abscess very quickly [Weber 2005]. I suspect that chewing on a few raw cashew nuts before going to bed would almost eliminate all tooth decay.

It is desirable to have variety in the vegetables, as almost every plant has a different mild poison or another and variety prevents difficulty from any one of them. For instance parsnip root and diseased celery have a phototoxic poison [Ivie], poisons in soy beans have damaging affect [shttp://nutritionwonderland.com/2010/03/the-protein-problem-eating-healthy-while-making-the-least-ecological-impact-soy/] (also see this extensive discussion [http://www.westonaprice.org/soy-alert.html]) - and capsaicin in chili pepper placed on the nerves surrounding the insulin cells in mice kills the nerves [http://www.canada.com/nationalpost/news/story.html?id=a042812e-492c-4f07-8245-8a598ab5d1bf&k=63970] and may cause type I diabetes [Weber 2008] (see chapter 6). Each plant family is usually different from the others. Therefore, it is important to vary your menu. If you concentrate on one particular plant, you may find yourself in the embarrassing position of the man who turned orange from eating too many tomatoes and carrots, or have a vital food element tied up in the digestive tract as the oxalic acid in spinach and rhubarb is alleged to do to calcium, have your thyroid secretion decreased by something in canola oil, turnips, peanuts, soy nuts, pine nuts, uncooked, unfermented cruciferous vegetables (such as cabbage, broccoli, kale, and cauliflower [http://www.ithyroid.com/goitrogens.htm] or, much worse, to be badly sickened by alkaloids as the poor people in India are sometimes when they eat only a local wild pea during a famine. Most of these toxic substances are only mildly toxic and present in small amounts in cultivated plants so variety should solve the problem satisfactorily for edible plants for most people. You can see which foods belong to which families in order to rotate and maximize the advantage at; this site [http://www.mall-net.com/mcs/rotate.html]. One way to achieve variety is to find recipes for good tasting mixtures of food. You may see a link to a trail mix recipe in this site [http://www.fugitt.com/trailmix.htm]. A fringe benefit is that mixtures of vegetables almost always taste better than individual vegetables, in my opinion. Soup is an especially tasty way to eat vegetables, but do not discard the boil water because it contains potassium, etc. A recipe for a Korean blend of vegetables called Kimchi similar to sauerkraut may be seen here [http://www.treelight.com/health/nutrition/UltimateKimchi.html]. Be sure to go very easy on the salt though, or use potassium salt. Another recipe, for a [http://www.vsh.org/Fruit_Smoothie4.htm] blended vegetable drink which Harris calls a 'smoothie" is here * [http://www.vsh.org/smoothies.htm]. His suggestion to use a 50 milligram zinc supplement is very dangerous and should not be taken though, because excess zinc interferes with copper.

MEAT TOXINS

There are no toxic meats in normal commerce, so that variety in meat is probably not essential to take care of the above circumstance about poisons. It has been proposed that red meat is unhealthy, but this is an invalid myth, so people with adequate kidneys or do not suffer from hemochromatosis (inability to excrete iron) can eat large amounts of red meat safely. Eating red meat as being unhealthy is an incorrect perception probably produced by charred meat producing cancer causing chemicals and processed meats containing numerous poisonous additives. There are tribes in Africa whose members make meat a major part of their diet in which degenerative diseases are very rare [http://www.westonaprice.org/traditional-diets/623-out-of-africa.html]. Tribes that ate both meat and plant food were healthiest, so meat should be acceptable nutritionally to most who do not have quasi religious aversion to it. Epidemiological studies have linked red meat to rheumatoid arthritis [Pattison]. I suspect that the largest part of this correlation arises from a tendency for arthritics to be more allergic to some proteins, so this should disappear when the rheumatoid arthritis disappears from adequate potassium.

Most of the chickens are treated with an arsenic compound to kill intestinal parasites. This is a bad idea . However, the amounts of arsenic in the meat is probably too small to cause a serious health problem. Many poultry farms feed the birds salt water fish, which no doubt gives them tiny mounts of mercury. Chicken bones contain fluoride. You may be tempted to chew them because of their calcium content. This is not a good way to get calcium or phosphorus.

Many sausages, cold cuts, and hot dogs contain nitrates. It is my understanding that unprocessed meat is free of any chemicals.

An exception to poison in unprocessed meat is fish. Salt water fish can

contain unacceptable amounts of mercury [http://www.cfsan.fda.gov/~frf/
sea-mehg.html]. Large fish high in the food chain such as tuna are said to
be the highest in mercury. N-acetylcysteine (NAC) has been proposed as a
chelator of methylmercury for eliminating it from the body and as a test for
methylmercury load without bad side effects [Aremu]. Phytyc acid (inositol
hexaphosphate or IP6) in rice bran has been proposed as a potent chelator of
mercury, especially the extract. It has no bad side effects other than to prevent
some absorption of some essential mineral elements.

Tropical fish contain ciguatera toxin. This ciguatera is a poison of many
carbon rings generated by algae, which toxin can not be degraded by heat and
which is thought to bind to sodium cell wall pumps. It remains in the body for
a long time. It gives symptoms similar to chronic fatigue syndrome (CFS, ME,
or CFIDS). Mannitol has been proposed as a treatment [Karlin]. Since fish
migrate and in addition are transported all over the world, eating oceanic fish
(especially large reef fish) or pigs or chickens (it is said that chickens receive only
2% fishmeal) fed such fish may not be worth the risk even for healthy people
(Tyson Inc. claims no use of fish. Keep in mind that corporate procedures
sometimes change). I suspect that cod-liver oil is safe since it is a northern fish and
is a good source of vitamin D and omega 3 oil. Fish oils are safe from mercury,
since they contain only minute amounts of mercury [Foran] [http://arpa.
allenpress.com/arpaonline/?request=get-abstract&doi=10,1043%2F1543-
2165(2003)127%3C1603:MOMLIC%3E2.0.CO%3B2]. A recurrence of
neurological symptoms from ciguatera may be brought on by consumption
of alcohol (probably not the alcohol itself, but poisons associated with it) or
certain foods such as other fish, fish-flavored food products, meat such as
chicken and pork , and peanut butter or nut oils.

Another exception can be eating shellfish. There are two algae that have
a poison not degradable by heat that are filtered by shellfish. They produce
diseases called paralytic shellfish poisoning and paralytic shellfish poisonings
are present throughout the world when the appropriate bloom materializes
[Silver]. There is hope that they will become forestalled in the future by
development of robots that can detect the DNA of the poisonous algae and
monitor the bay water.

The next four chapters will explore the affects of a potassium deficiency on
heart disease, high blood pressure, rheumatoid arthritis, gout, and diabetes.

CHAPTER 3
HEART DISEASE AND HYPERTENSION

SUMMARY

It has been proven beyond any doubt that a potassium deficiency will cause heart disease in the presence of adequate vitamin B-1 by epidemiological surveys and numerous experiments on animals [Rubini]. Experiments on people are not possible because heart disease is very dangerous. The dangerous interaction between potassium and vitamin B-1, the affect of magnesium on the heart by way of potassium, the effects from magnesium as the orotate or the taurate on the heart, the invalidity of the cholesterol hypothesis, and the dependence of at least one of the forms of high blood pressure on chloride are discussed.

It has been proven beyond any doubt that a potassium deficiency will cause heart disease (death of heart cells) in the presence of adequate vitamin B-1 by epidemiological surveys and numerous experiments on animals [Rubini]. Experiments on people are not possible because heart disease is very dangerous.

Potassium has been used in heart disease therapy since 1930 [Sampson]. If the heart disease is the so called "wet" heart disease as associated with beri-beri (vitamin B-1 or thiamine deficiency) , potassium supplements will dangerously aggravate the situation [Mineno][Gould]. Therefore it is very important to know which kind of heart disease it is. If potassium supplements are given during the wet heart disease of vitamin B-1 deficiency (beri-beri), it has been proven that the heart disease is made much worse [Mineno] [Gould]. Wet heart disease of vitamin B-1 deficiency (beri-beri) is impossible if potassium is also deficient [Folis]. Instead a muscular atrophy similar to that from vitamin E deficiency appears [Hove][Blahd]. During a vitamin B-1 deficiency the heart loses potassium [Mineno]. This may be why heart damage in vitamin B-1 deficiency resembles that in a potassium deficiency. It is obvious that if potassium supplements are given, it is very important that the vitamin B-1 intake must be adequate at the same time, because the damage to the heart from vitamin B-1 deficiency is only possible when potassium is adequate. Even if people are eating foods adequate in vitamin B-1 they could still possibly have a problem with vitamin B-1 deficiency if they are also eating foods which have sulfites in them such as wine, vinegar, beer, bottled lemon juice, and some dried fruits (see these sites' appendix for a list of food containing sulfites [http://edis.ifas.ufl.edu/FY731] and [http://www.readingtarget.com/nosulfites/knowing.htm]), because sulfites degrade vitamin B-1 in the intestines [Amerine] [Fitzhugh]. Such foods are wine, vinegar, pickles, olives, salad dressing, canned clams, fresh, frozen, canned, or dried shrimp, frozen lobster, scallops, dried cod, gelatin, pectin jelling agents, cornstarch, modified food starch, spinach pasta, gravies, hominy, breadings, batters, noodle/rice mixes, shredded coconut, vegetable juice, canned vegetables (including potatoes), pickled vegetables (including sauerkraut), dried vegetables, instant mashed potatoes, frozen potatoes, potato salad, corn syrup, maple syrup, fruit toppings, and high-fructose syrups such as corn syrup and pancake syrup, instant tea, liquid tea concentrates, beer, bottled lemon juice, some baked goods, and some dried fruits or eat unfortified refined grains.

Using diuretics can cause loss of vitamin B-1 [Suter]. [http://www.ncbi.nlm.nih.gov/entrez/query.fcgi?itool=abstractplus&db=pubmed&cmd=Retrieve&dopt=abstractplus&list_uids-11127971].

There is something in tea leaves that antagonizes vitamin B-1 [http://www.ncbi.nlm.nih.gov/entrez/query.fcgi?db=pubmed&cmd=Retrieve&dopt=AbstractPlus&list_uids=2005509&query_hl=7&itool=pubmed_DocSum] possibly thiaminase, an enzyme that degrades vitamin B-1.

A folate deficiency can inhibit vitamin B-1 absorption [Thomson]

The diet can vary widely as to vitamin B-1 [Dept. of Health]. One symptom of a vitamin B-1 deficiency is lactic acid acidosis [Romanski]. Also, the symptoms of a vitamin B-1 deficiency can materialize even if vitamin B-1 is adequate if magnesium is deficient, as in Crohn's disease [http://www.ncbi.nlm.nih.gov/entrez/query.fcgi?cmd=Retrieve&db=PubMed&list_uids=4050546&dopt=Citation][Dyckner, Nyhlin, Wester].

As a result, one third of the people admitted to a New Jersey hospital were low in vitamin B-1.

Even in the more likely circumstance that the heart disease is largely a potassium deficiency or aggravated by one, potassium should be used with great caution shortly after an attack. Even though the cellular content is low, and some heart cells are actually dying for lack of potassium, the plasma content can be too high [Flear][Hurley][White] and so supplements can be dangerous. Raab, in a comprehensive review, suggests that dying cells may not be able to reabsorb potassium during the acute phases and thus cause death from this and the adjacent hyperkalemia (high blood potassium). He suggests adopting the words "disionic cardiopathy" in order to avoid the semantic confusion and invalidity inherent in such words as "coronary heart disease" [Raab]. It is imperative to keep potassium intake from supplements adequate though, because a deficiency causes the heart to lose force [Abbrecht]. The way some doctors in the world get around the impasse is to administer the potassium in conjunction with glucose sugar and insulin [Sodi-Pollares] [Iosava][Landman][Hjermann][LaMarche]. Thus much of the potassium enters the cell to be tied up with glycogen (animal starch). This is called a "polarizing solution" or "GIK" (glucose-insulin-potassium). It is fairly affective although it must not be used during the "wet" heart disease of beri-beri (vitamin B-1 deficiency) as discussed above. The insulin may be also speeding movement of potassium across the cell wall because of its affect on a glucose - potassium pump [Lundman]. The insulin response is similar in both normal and potassium deficient animals. They therefore conclude that potassium deficient animals secrete less insulin [Mondon] [Heianza]. This procedure was originally proposed by Laborit and Huguenard [Laborit & Huguenard]] in France and Sodi-Pollares in Mexico in 1962 [Rackley]. This therapy benefits some patients but is unpredictable [Thadani][Fletcher], probably because the "wet" heart disease of beri-beri (vitamin B-1 deficiency) is sometimes involved or because some other deficiency predominates. This procedure has fallen into disfavor but is now being restudied.

MAGNESIUM

Magnesium is the second most prevalent cation in the body's cells. About sixty % is found in the bones with the remainder in the cells and one % in the blood plasma. Wheat germ is the richest source. Taking large amounts of extra calcium interferes with magnesium absorption.

The unpredictability for heart disease may be also partly because some of the heart disease is caused or accentuated by magnesium [http://www.krispin.com/magnes.html].. deficiency[http://www.krispin.com/magnes.html]. It has been proposed that most heart disease is a magnesium deficiency. I suspect that this perception arises because much of the affect of magnesium is operating through the potassium physiology. For instance, it is thought that the reduction of magnesium is what causes the association of potassium with high blood pressure (hypertension) by virtue of the affect of magnesium on the power of the potassium-sodium pumps. Potassium depletion causes salt sensitive high blood pressure (hypertension) in Dahl rats. High blood pressure is an important risk factor in stroke. Even so, a study found that only 400 milligrams per day of potassium supplements caused a 40% reduction in stroke mortality. This effect was independent of other dietary variables in the study, including the intake of calories, fat, protein, fiber, calcium, magnesium (this last further hinting that magnesium is acting by its affect on potassium), and alcohol. The affect was also independent of known or suspected cardiovascular risk factors, including age, sex, blood pressure, blood cholesterol level, obesity, fasting blood glucose level, and cigarette smoking [Khaw]. The article in this URL explores the above and potassium affects on calcium, magnesium, and phosphate excretions [http://www.lef.org/prod_hp/abstracts/potassiumabs.html#5].

It has been proposed that most heart disease is a magnesium deficiency. I suspect that this perception arises because much of the affect of magnesium is operating through the potassium physiology. For instance, it is thought that the reduction of magnesium causes potassium to be absorbed or reabsorbed with less efficiency and thus cause high blood pressure (hypertension) by virtue of the affect of magnesium on the power of the potassium-sodium pumps as elaborated above.

Six months are required of magnesium supplements before complete normalization of pumps [http://www.lef.org/prod_hp/abstracts/potassiumabs.html#26]. This may be part of the reason why magnesium did not seem to have a close affect on potassium supplementation above. The richest sources of magnesium in food are green vegetables because magnesium is contained in chlorophyll.

Whang and Flink have proposed to add magnesium to GIK (glucose-insulin-potassium) and calling the therapy MAGIK [Whang and Flink]. Also see this site about magnesium [http://www.mgwater.com/cardio.shtml]. Usually magnesium should be part of heart disease treatment. Its efficacy in heart disease has been documented by numerous studies, including [Schecter]. Probably reasonable, recommended amounts of magnesium supplements would never be harmful to the heart, but I have no sure evidence. It is very affective in atrial fibrillation or excessive heart beats. Magnesium lowered average heart rate by 25 beats per minute more (130 to 105 for the drug digoxin versus 130 to 80 for magnesium plus digoxin) than the savings from digoxin alone [Brodsky] in 60% of patients. In other words, magnesium helped those patients 'save' 36,000 heart beats per day over what they would have saved with the drug alone. The following referenced experiments involve low serum potassium, in which potassium could not be increased in the body with 1,000 milligrams of potassium supplement without magnesium [Kohvacca] [http://www.mgwater.com/schroll.shtml],

One person reports getting red cell magnesium up to normal with magnesium orotate and Epsom magnesium sulfate foot baths every other day, along with a choline citrate supplement in the hope the latter helps with absorption. Magnesium as the orotate (orotate is pyrimidinecarboxylic acid, also known as orotic acid or vitamin B13, Animal Galactose Factor, Oro, Orodin, Oropur, Orotonin, Oroturic, Orotyl, or whey factor.) has been shown to be more readily absorbed than as the carbonate [Schlebusch]. Orotate is not usually recognized as a vitamin. It is manufactured in the body by intestinal flora. Athletes had their swimming, cycling, and running times decreased in the magnesium-orotate group compared with the controls and their insulin system markedly affected [Golf]. This may have been partly due to the orotate itself, because orotate is incorporated into RNA, enabled by biotin [http://www.jbc.org/cgi/reprint/245/21/5600.pdf]. People with coronary heart disease had their exercise ability significantly increased by magnesium orotate [Geiss]. Orotic acid is not necessarily always good in excess since it is said to bind zinc to a non-biologically active state and can damage the liver, but the 50 to 100 milligrams that have been recommended by some should be safe. Sources of orotate are whey, yogurt, beetroot, carrots, and Jerusalem artichoke, but not human milk.

TAURINE

Taurate has been proposed as the best magnesium supplement [McCarty 1996]. Taurine or 2-aminoethanesulfonic acid is an acidic chemical substance sulfonated rather than carboxylated found in high abundance in the tissues of many animals (metazoa), especially sea animals. Taurine is also found in plants, fungi, and some bacterial species, but in far less abundance. It is an amine with a sulfonic acid functional group, but it is not an amino acid in the biological sense, not being one of the twenty protein-forming compounds encoded by the universal genetic code. Small polypeptides have been identified as containing taurine, but to date there has been no report of a transfer RNA that is specifically charged with taurine [all taurine information above from Wikipedia]. Taurine is essential to babies.

It has been found that supplements of the amino acid, taurine, will restore the abnormal electrocardiogram present during a potassium deficiency by an unknown mechanism [Eby], but also see Dumaine [Dumaine]. This information has been used in several case histories by George Eby to control a long standing type of cardiac arrhythmia called pre atrial contractions

(PACs), a benign but irritating and nerve racking heart problem, with 2.5 grams of taurine with each meal. In animal or clinical studies, taurine lowers elevated blood pressure, retards cholesterol-induced atherogenesis, prevents arrhythmias and stabilizes platelets--effects parallel to those of magnesium [McCarty 1996].

Taurine is said to be low in the diets of vegetarians. The 2.5 grams recommended by the American Heart Association causes diarrhea in some people and should be reduced in those cases. Taurine has been used for high blood pressure, migraine headache, high cholesterol, epilepsy, macular degeneration, Alzheimer's disease, liver disorders, alcoholism, cystic fibrosis, and depression. Keep in mind that some people may have a genetic defect that limits the amount of taurine tolerated and that adequate molybdenum may be desirable. Also taurine may make a copper deficiency worse based on a single case history, so adequate copper may be necessary [Brien Quirk, private communication].

OTHER HEART DISEASE UNPREDICTABILITY

Part of the unpredictability of heart disease may arise because of the dependence of the sodium/potassium pump on inositol [Charalampous] [Greene](a B complex vitamin or myoinositol), or because of unpredictable huge sodium, chloride, or phosphate (from soft drinks) excess. There is 100% mortality in heart attack during potassium deficiency in the presence of excess phosphate [Selye], for instance from soft drinks (especially colas [Hall]). It has been suggested that diabetics should not be treated with polarizing solution [Rackley]. However, a recent experiment has indicated improved results post operatively using GIK polarizing solution (glucose-insulin-potassium) for coronary operations [Szabo]. If whatever nutritional imbalance is not addressed correctly the prognosis is poor for heart disease patients. Potassium is prescribed for 40% of heart disease patients. This prescription percentage should probably be much higher, but not so high as to include patients with beri-beri (vitamin B-1 deficiency). Only 50% of one group survived after 5 years. Anyone suffering from a vitamin B-1 deficiency would be especially at severe risk from potassium supplements if animal experiments are an indication [Follis]. Anxiety often attends a potassium deficiency [Davis], probably because of low aldosterone affect on the nervous system, so this may serve as a clue as to which kind of heart disease is involved and would bear investigation. The only sure way to determine cell potassium is with a whole body scintillation counter, although plasma potassium much below about 4.0 meq/L (milliequivalents per liter) would be a strong indication. The risk of heart disease does not change significantly when the mean serum potassium content of patient groups changes between 4.1 milliequivalents (meq) per liter and 5.3 meq [Walsh], so while it is no doubt desirable to attain the normal 4.8 milligrams per liter in blood (or possibly a little less than 4.8 if correctly measured), the situation does not seem to be desperately dangerous above 4.0. One exception to this would be people who have rheumatoid arthritis, whose platelets release some potassium into the plasma upon blood being drawn [Ifudu] and thus give an incorrect reading. There is also a new procedure using neutron bombardment of cells [http://www.exatest.com/Research.htm] that may yet show promise.

In any case, there is no good substitute for whole, unprocessed foods with lots of vegetables [http://www.findarticles.com/cf_0/m0887/2_22/98171061/p1/article.jhtml] either alone or with some supplements to prevent heart disease in the first place. Vegetables and fruit have been established by epidemiological studies to protect against heart disease [http://jn.nutrition.org/cgi/content/abstract/136/10/2588] and in this survey [http://www.ajcn.org/cgi/content/abstract/76/1/93] and also by experiments on mice [http://jn.nutrition.org/cgi/content/abstract/136/7/1886].

Serum potassium of 3.5 meq per liter or less increases problems in heart surgery and doubles arrhythmias. Below 3.3 meq doubles the necessity of resuscitation. These figures should be higher for people with rheumatoid arthritis because they get unusually high readings, especially of serum rather than plasma, as mentioned above.

Judging by the statistics associated with heart disease therapy, potassium and magnesium [Bajusz p 168] must be playing dominant roles in a majority of current cases, because potassium, whether in polarizing solutions, GIK (glucose-insulin-potassium), as potassium chloride [Chang], or as potassium and magnesium aspartate [Laborit][Classen] causes a considerable reduction in mortality in the USA and especially abroad. Kadaner found that 3,000 to 4,000 milligrams of potassium chloride per day for 3-4 weeks prevented or considerably alleviated vascular crises. Most showed a decrease in blood pressure of 30-40 mm of mercury when taken with reserpine, hydrochlorothiazide, and some other drugs, which by themselves did not give such an effect [Kadaner]. Also people working in potash mines have a lower heart disease rate than others [Waxweiler]. Elderly heart disease patients given potassium supplements usually show an increase in whole body potassium [Potter]. It is impossible to cause heart disease experimentally by any known poison unless the potassium intake is also restricted or the kidneys destroyed [Prioreschi]. The lack of total body potassium parallels the severity of the disease [Pierson].

Wine has been correlated with low heart disease rates. I suspect that this is because wine contains a poison that interferes with potassium excretion [McDonald] or perhaps because sulfites, in most wine, destroys vitamin

B-1. If so, getting enough potassium in the diet would be a much superior strategy for achieving this result for several reasons, even if the wine has been fermented without sulfur dioxide.

Vitamin C and vitamin E supplements produce significant reductions in the incidence of heart trouble. Indeed adequate amounts of all the essential nutrients by increasing general health no doubt have significant affects on all various kinds of heart trouble such as plaque build up, arrhythmias, aneurysms, and death of cells. If you insist on eating only whole foods, most of the essential nutrients other than vitamin D, iodide, and, to some extent, vitamin C, will be almost always at least reasonably adequate.

High blood pressure can have damaging affects on the kidneys and to some extent on the heart, chocolate has the affect of lowering blood pressure somewhat [http://www.nutritionevidencelibrary.com/evidence.cfm?evidence_summary_id=250220&highlight=hypertension&home=1] . There is some evidence that garlic can lower high blood pressure.

CHOLESTEROL

Heart disease as caused by blockage of blood vessels by cholesterol has been attributed to cholesterol in the diet. While excessive intakes may contribute to this blockage slightly, a disruption of normal cholesterol synthesis in the body must be the primary cause and in any case adequate potassium has a protective affect [Young]. Cholesterol in the diet has only risen from 683 milligrams in 1900 to 734 per day in 1961 and Masai tribesmen have low blood cholesterol in spite of high unsaturated fat in the diet [Brown]. A copper deficiency has the characteristic of increasing cholesterol in the blood stream [Allen]. A histidine induced cholesterol rise is abolished by copper supplements [Harvey]. It has been suggested that a high zinc to copper intake ratio is an important part of this [Klevay 1978]. The rise in cholesterol and triglycerides has been attributed to a 40% or more reduction in lipoprotein lipase. This is a copper containing enzyme. This may be an adaptation to provide extra cholesterol for lining the arteries with deposits in order to help protect them against rupture by decreasing their internal diameter, for the stress on the walls is directly proportional to the radius. Whatever the evolutionary stimulus is, copper deficiency is a much more plausible explanation of high serum cholesterol than any difference in cholesterol intake, because the body can synthesize its own cholesterol. No enzyme system has been linked to this phenomenon yet with certainty to my knowledge. However, the reduction of lipoprotein lipase during copper deficiency has been proposed [Lau]. Non ceruloplasmin copper is said to signal the increase of cholesterol [Harvey]. Cholesterol lowering drugs have not prevented deaths and the cholesterol level is normal in the average heart attack victim. For some side effects of cholesterol lowering drugs see links in this site [http://www.thincs.org/unpublic.htm].

ADDITIONAL AFFECTERS

Because the clearance of blood through the liver is reduced in heart disease, partly because of lack of exercise, aldosterone builds up [Cope]. Aldosterone is normally constantly destroyed by liver enzymes as fast as it is produced [Messerli]. As a result it is difficult to restore the body's potassium with food alone [Howard] [White] [Liddle] [Randall]. If supplements are prescribed, probably the safest way to take them would be between meals, in small doses, and dissolved in juice. It is possible to largely restore the body's potassium with potassium chloride supplements in two weeks or so [Conway]. Using potassium chloride should be reasonably safe even for those who have high blood pressure because potassium chloride had almost the same affect in lowering blood pressure as potassium bicarbonate [He]. It is the chloride in salt that produces high blood pressure, though,, not the sodium, although the presence of sodium is necessary [Boegshold]. Potassium is not affective in lowering blood pressure in the presence of a high sodium chloride intake [http://www.foodbase.org.uk/results.php?f_category_id=&f_report_id=74]. There is a close epidemiological relation to salt intake in various tribes and a rise in blood pressure incidence with age [http://physrev.physiology.org/cgi/reprint/85/2/679.pdf].

Also it would be wise to receive as much potassium as possible from food. In addition, it is probably advantageous not to supplement one's diet with sodium and chloride from salt, phosphate from soft drinks, or vitamin B1 (thiamin). Death of heart cells from a potassium deficiency is prevented by a thiamin deficiency [Follis], so supplementing vitamin B-1 prematurely could be dangerous unless the heart disease was established as the "wet" heart disease of beri beri (vitamin B-1 deficiency) as discussed above. When both potassium and vitamin B-1 are deficient lesions of the muscles occur instead similar to muscular dystrophy (potassium is low in muscular dystrophy cases [Blahd]). The danger might be especially present if you have been imbibing wine, vinegar or beer fermented with sulfur dioxide or eating fruit dried with sulfur dioxide because sulfur dioxide and sulfites rapidly destroy vitamin B-1 from the pH of the intestines [Amerine p487] [Fitzhugh]. Some of the symptoms of a magnesium deficiency are also muted by a simultaneous vitamin B-1 deficiency [Hokawa], possibly because of the affect of magnesium deficiency on potassium absorption.

Of course, the most affective lifetime strategy would be to get all the potassium and other nutrients that were originally in the food, no huge excesses, and to eat, drink or smoke no poisons in the first place. Then you will not usually be likely to get a serious heart condition in which you must make such dangerous, expensive, and time consuming compromises and unnecessarily tie up medical facilities.

CHAPTER 4
RHEUMATOID ARTHRITIS

SUMMARY

It is my contention that potassium deficiency is either causing, or permitting, rheumatoid arthritis, Symptoms of rheumatoid arthritis are discussed. The symptoms are very technical and lay readers may want to study those parts. Evidence for potassium's involvement is presented. Various treatments for rheumatoid arthritisusing potassium are presented. Symptoms of a potassium deficiency are described.

There is not any indication in the literature that potassium has ever been tried by scientists as a cure for arthritis. A rather exhaustive search of the medical literature has failed to disclose any experiment. This includes Exerpta Medica 1947 to 1974, and a computer search by the Central Library of the American Medical Association from 1965 on back. In addition no search of mine since has revealed an experiment in the literature. It is only recently that a clinical trial has been performed by Rastmanesh with very encouraging results [Rastmanesh]. Even in the present, extensive books on arthritis fail to even mention potassium [Koopman] [Sobel]. Even extensive books on electrolytes fail to mention rheumatoid arthritis [Halpern] [Narins].

Arthritis or rheumatism is a major crippling disease in America. At least 2.1 million people in the USA have rheumatoid arthritis. A Brazilian study indicates that one half a per cent have rheumatoid arthritis as opposed to about 4% for osteoarthritis in that country, [http://listserv.nodak.edu/scripts/wa.exe?A2=ind0403A&L=co-cure&P=R5826&D=0] and 2% for rheumatoid arthritis has been estimated for the USA [Rasch]. The CDC says that at least 65 billion dollars are lost each year for medical costs and loss of productivity, but that figure does not a even begin to measure degradation of quality of life. There is an estimate that individual costs average $5700 per year and present estimates for direct and indirect costs add up to 128 billion dollars. [http://vitalvotes.com/blogs/public_blog/America-s-Arthritis-Costs-Skyrocket-Along-With-Obesity/4001.aspx]. It causes more disability in its victims than heart disease [http://www3.interscience.wiley.com/journal/121425832/abstract]. Two thirds of the victims are women, most of them over 45 [Rodman]. The terrible pains associated with rheumatoid arthritis, reminiscent of and similar to the medieval torture racks must surely be among the top causes of contemporary misery. These pains, along with the actual physical disability, weak joints, loss of energy, and other systemic symptoms [http://www.nlm.nih.gov/medlineplus/ency/article/000431.htm#causesAndRisk] that accompany them, cause an enormous loss of productivity. Half the patients will stop working within 10 years. Both kinds o arthritis are probably a considerable part of the cause of increasing welfare roles. Even industrial accidents are related to this monstrous and onerous burden that society carries. Small jolts and falls that should do little more than bring out some colorful language results in loss of hours and even months. It is more than just the loss of time itself. It is also the super caution that blocks even fairly healthy people from making fast, risky moves when they see some of the debacles their friends get into. It is well worth getting rid of.

Nor is rheumatoid arthritis confined to North America. Countries at such extremes of latitude as Finland and Jamaica have even higher rates than we do [Kellgren]. The simple life is not any guarantee against misery either, nor is a simple life a guarantee of good nutrition. The Masai tribesmen of Africa have high rates [Best p768], perhaps because of high perspiration potassium loss and eating a diet low in vegetables. Political or economic ideologies are not barriers. Rheumatoid arthritis is present in Russia, is also present in nomadic hunters, and cave men, cave bears, and ancient Egyptians are thought to have had it [Bach][Crain], although Rothschild believes it first started among Tennessee Indians 4000 years ago and spread from there [http://mcclungmuseum.utk.edu/research/renotes/rn-05txt.htm]. It shows no obvious clear association with any culture even though it is very variable, with very low rates in tribes near the Masai (including villages in Nigeria [Silman]) and Laplanders near the Finns in Finland, as well as insane people in Massachusetts [Allander p260] and an absence of arthritis on the island of Triton da Cuhna [Kellgren]. There is no evidence of rheumatoid arthritis among early Australian aborigines [Roberts-Thompson] or among Eskimos [Phelps]. The rates are very variable within regions of North America, within ethnic and economic groups, and age groups. 15.2% of white people,. 15.5%

of black people, 11.3% of Hispanics, and 7.3% of Asian Pacific islanders have rheumatic conditions [Helmick] (but not all rheumatoid).

SYMPTOMS OF RHEUMATOID ARTHRITIS

A considerably large fraction of the people who have pains in the joints have them because of rheumatoid arthritis. The pains usually strike first in the outer joints like wrists, carpels, fingers on both sides, or joints with a history of injury. If a patient completely lacks hand and wrist pain involvement, a diagnosis of rheumatoid arthritis is doubtful. Load bearing joints are also vulnerable. Joints look much different in rheumatoid than they do in osteoarthritis. The pain is most likely in the early morning. It is often accompanied by stiffness. It is not to be assumed that the disease is localized because the pain is, Rheumatoid arthritis is present throughout the body and can affect kidneys, pericardium of the heart, and connecting tissue (mesenchyme tissue) [Strukov][Ropes]. It is a disease largely associated with humans [LaMont-Havers], probably partly because animals can not talk (or in the case of rodents possibly because they make no use of cortisol (see the cortisol chapter 12 for further discussion of this last), but I suspect primarily because animals usually do not have access to refined food low in potassium.

Rheumatoid arthritis has few externally observable symptoms, especially in early stages. There are no known consistent biochemical changes in rheumatoid arthritis except a lower cellular potassium content than normal [LaCelle][Sambrook], and a somewhat higher plasma copper content along with a protein which binds the copper in the serum [Schubert]. However there are reports of some changes that show up in a high proportion of arthritics. There have been reports of low salivary potassium (the only consistent difference from normal they found) [Syrjanen], low serum potassium [Cockel], calcium, phosphorus, lysozyme, and IgA peptide in the saliva of juvenile arthritics [Siamopoulou et al] (which form of arthritis could be similar to the adult form). The immune peptide hormones, IL18, MIF, CCL2, CCL3, CCL11, CXCL9 and CXCL10, are statistically higher in juvenile arthritis [Jager]. The activity of sodium/potassium ATPase is lower during rheumatoid arthritis in the erythrocyte (red blood cell) membrane [Masoon-Yasinzai] and lower than in normal, osteoarthritis, or gout [Testa]. Autoreactive T cells from patients with type-1 diabetes mellitus or arthritis are mainly CD4(+)CCR7(-)CD45RA(-) affecter memory T cells (T(EM) cells) with elevated Kv1.3 potassium channel expression [Beeton]. The steroid hormone dehydroepiandrosterone sulfate (DHEA) is statistically lower in rheumatoid arthritics [Dessein] as is cortisol, pregnanediol and basal DHEAS [Imrich], even though ACTH is higher, as is aldosterone [Khetagurova]. The aldosterone being higher suggests that there is something besides the low potassium itself that is involved in the cause of rheumatoid arthritis because aldosterone stimulates excretion of potassium and has a positive feedback. See chapter 11, History of Arthritis Research, for some speculation from the past as to what that something might be.

There is different spectrum of amino acids in the blood serum of arthritics [Trang]. The ratio of IL6 peptide immune hormone to cortisol is statistically correlated to number of swollen joints and low grip strength [Straub]. There has been an effort to use changes in some of the body's other proteins in diagnosis, but with limited success so far, although some of the other rheumatic diseases can be almost diagnosed from blood proteins alone [Waller]. As nearly as I can tell most of the above seemed to be the consensus for rheumatoid arthritis at the 1982 Pan American Conference on Arthritis and largely remains so today. There are significant correlations between IgM, RF, and IgA immune proteins and a higher disease activity [Chen] but the correlations are not perfect and IgM RF and C reactive protein are commonly used in modern testing labs. There is lower glycosylation of immune peptides (addition of sugar molecules) during rheumatoid arthritis [Axford]. I do not know what the significance of this is although addition of sugars may prevent the peptides from being normally active. C3 and C4 compliments are said to be the best of the other discriminators [Sari, et al]. In epithelial sodium channels, alpha and beta subunits are higher than normal in rheumatoid arthritis but not present in osteoarthritis [Trujillo, et al]. There is high activity of collagenase and elastase in the synovial fluid of patients with rheumatoid arthritis, which is about 30 times higher than that found in the synovial fluid of patients with osteoarthritis [Bazzichi]. Rheumatoid arthritis sometimes has fatigue associated with it. The settling rate of red blood cells (erythrocytes) is said to be different in rheumatoid arthritis [from a dead URL], but is very variable and unreliable. Adrenomedulin, a peptide hormone, is three times higher in synovial fluid in rheumatoid arthritis than it is in osteoarthritis [Matsushita]. Also there is a high level of human leucocyte antigen in saliva of rheumatoid arthritis and lupus erythmatosis, and none in normal saliva [Adamashvili].

In the past rheumatoid arthritis was associated with old age in people's minds and there was a tendency to suffer it stoically as inevitable. It is a serious disease, though, with a much reduced life span and a 27% mortality at ten years. While the medical profession has intellectually abandoned an assumption that only people in old age are affected, many laymen still assume this is the case. The concept that this is "old age" is pervasive, even creeping into common cultural media as modern as "Star Trek". This is not to indicate that the victims did not often attempt to do something. Rheumatoid arthritis has a long history of quack nostrums and screwball procedures. These quack remedies were assisted by the numerous spontaneous remissions that occur with rheumatoid arthritis or by pain deadening chemicals. It was not necessary to cure everyone, since those who were "cured" were very grateful and those who were not were fatalistic, since their doctors could do nothing either. See chapter 11 for a discussion of the history of rheumatoid arthritis research,

POTASSIUM IN THE ETIOLOGY OF RHEUMATOID ARTHRITIS

It is my suspicion that rheumatoid arthritis is a potassium deficiency that makes it impossible for a cell to get rid of bacteria that invades the interior of the cell like a virus does. I suspect that some poison or some infections or decline in kidney function with age degrades our ability to concentrate potassium and thus makes it impossible to get adequate potassium from food from which almost every processing procedure removes potassium these days. Arthritics characteristically have poor nourishment [Morgan et al] [Stone] including magnesium [Kremer], which is necessary for potassium absorption. A poison that I suspect damages the kidneys in such a way as to prevent potassium retention, is the very poisonous bromine gas, since it probably affected me that way 60 years ago. It is possible that the glucocorticosteroid response modifying peptide hormone (GRMF) to be discussed in the cortisol chapter 12, may be the system involved in the case of infection triggers, because of cortisol's rise from endotoxin along with a possible inability for GRMF to block cortisol's action on potassium. Not much is known about GRMF's affect on physiological processes or how rheumatoid arthritis affects it.

The National Health and Nutrition Survey-III has determined that of 39,695 people selected, there were 840 who said they had been diagnosed with rheumatoid arthritis. Of these, 691 had their serum tested for potassium. Of that number 7.8% had less than 3.6 milliequivalents per liter, 34.7% between 3.6 and 4.0, 40.7% between 4.0 and 4.4, and 18.1% above 4.4. Therefore, only 18% appeared to be in the normal range. 4.8 is the value the body attempts to achieve. The samples were refrigerated and sent out to outside contract laboratories [NHANES-III]. Refrigerating blood increases the apparent amount when it is serum that is analyzed, especially if there is a delay in the analysis. In addition to that, rheumatoid arthritics lose potassium from the platelets as noted above. If some were misdiagnosed, had a remission since being diagnosed, or there was a longer than usual delay in analysis, it could account for the 18% seemingly normal. So that survey showed at least most arthritics low in serum potassium. Many others in the survey were low in potassium also. So, unless rheumatoid arthritis is caused by something besides a potassium deficiency and low potassium is either a symptom or an accentuating factor, those other survey people would have to have had rheumatoid arthritis as well. I believe that many people die of heart disease caused by a potassium deficiency (see chapter 3) without being arthritic, so, if so, the first part of that last statement must be in order. Also, in a group of tuberculosis patients medicated with capreomycin, 31% developed hypokalemia [Shin] and none of them had rheumatoid arthritis [Shin, private communication]. Tuberculosis is a mycoplasma bacteria, and mycoplasma has been suggested as causing rheumatoid arthritis, as mentioned in chapter 11. So perhaps that antibiotic solved the arthritis at the same time. In any case, a large proportion of arthritics, at least, are too low in potassium levels for sure, some dangerously low.

ARTHRITIS TREATMENTS WITH POTASSIUM

One technique, which seemed to have some success, was the use of spas. At least their popularity would seem to indicate some success. The Dead Sea water has a reputation for healing rheumatoid arthritis and has been successfully investigated with healing lasting up to three months [Sukenik]. It has about 5 times or so as much potassium chloride by weight as sodium chloride and an even greater amount of magnesium chloride by weight

One would think that warming the water high enough to open sweat gland pores would increase the speed of the affect if most of the potassium was entering through their mucous lining. That king-sized spa, the ocean, has been given credit for anti-arthritic tendencies also. This is plausible because the ocean contains potassium in about the same concentration as normal blood fluid. Sea mud is also given credit for curative properties [Veinpalu]. The spa at Bath, England, has potassium content less than one tenth that of ocean water [Riley]. If it is typical of spas, then unless they were drinking the water, it is hard to see how it could have helped there.

There have been closer associations with potassium. At one time sulfurated potash was used to combat rheumatoid arthritis [Osol p1092]. It is not surprising that it fell into disfavor associated with such a useless and poisonous anion. An anion is a negatively charged substance which neutralizes the positive charge of an ion such as potassium. The first person to definitively link potassium to rheumatoid arthritis in no uncertain terms was DeCoti-Marsh in a book published in England in 1957 [deCoti-Marsh]. He claimed numerous case histories. He recommended many anions to go with the potassium. His pioneering efforts enabled him to form a foundation currently active in England that encourages people to use potassium supplements in order to bring cell potassium up to normal and it has helped more than 3500 people [http://www.arthriticassociation.org.uk]. Recently potassium supplements in connection with drugs gave a good response in similar diseases [Casatta].

A successful technique was the raw vegetable diet described by Holbrook in Europe during the forties [Holbrook]. This diet became quite popular, even though most people must have found it fairly unpalatable. Eppinger hinted that the success of this diet might have been due to its high potassium content [Eppinger]. It might have become more popular if a recommendation to use fried vegetables, soup, or to drink the boil water had been made, which would have permitted the same potassium intake as raw. It would be a good idea to find out if vegetables being raw are additionally advantageous, especially since it has been found that cooking some food increases the growth rate of animals [http://www.unu.edu/unupress/unupbooks/80478e/80478E0j.htm], probably because interfering materials are destroyed in some of the vegetables by the cooking. This is something that would be especially important for children. There have been experiments with vegetarian diets in recent years but they have been changed merely by removing meat from the diet, not grains, which is probably why only moderate success has been attained [Hafstrom]. However, recently improvement has been noted using a diet that had increased amounts of vegetable juice and unpolished rice [Fujita]. There also has been a study that showed a strong negative correlation with cooked vegetables in Greece [Linos] and in Italy [[LaVecchia]. Dr. Saul has described a case in which vegetable juice and vegetables healed a woman. Kjeldsen-Kragh explored the affect of a vegetarian diet [Kjedsen-Kragh]. He found that fasting followed by a vegetarian diet has a favorable influence on disease activity in some patients with rheumatoid arthritis. This effect cannot be explained entirely by psychobiologic factors, immune suppression secondary to energy deprivation, changes in the plasma concentration of eicosanoid precursors, or changes in antibody activity against dietary antigens. Fasting should not be prolonged, or even attempted, because muscle wasting during rheumatoid arthritis is dangerous and weight reduction is not a factor in amelioration from vegetarian diets.

That diet is deeply involved in rheumatoid arthritis seems almost certain because when people migrate from areas with very low rheumatoid arthritis rates and start eating processed food, they come down with rheumatoid arthritis [http://www.drmcdougall.com/res_arthritis.html]. At the present time there are several books relating diet to arthritis. Jarvis stresses honey and vinegar in his book [Jarvis]. He instructed farmers to add potassium as apple cider vinegar to the rations of cows whose joints were swollen with arthritis and over the space of a year the enlarged joints returned to normal size and function. A farmer reported that 10 teaspoons of apple cider vinegar in water cured all the lameness and pain of his arthritis in one month's time.

Since honey is extremely low in potassium, the honey part would be counter productive. The vinegar could be very beneficial if well fed people are failing to metabolize [Winegrad] all of the acetate ion in vinegar or the acetate is being excreted by the kidneys before it has a chance to enter the cells, because the acid hydrogen ion interferes with potassium at the excretion site. I know of no tests reported in the literature testing this concept. Jarvis hints at other dietary changes also, which if followed, would increase potassium intake inadvertently. Kombucha, a vinegar like ferment, is said to be helpful for arthritis. Dong and Banks prescribe a diet free of chemicals, milk, meat and sugar, and low in fat [Dong]. If his diet were followed it would definitely increase potassium intake, especially since he stresses unprocessed vegetables. However, he attributes its success to freedom from allergens and chemicals, so that philosophically he tends to be in the same general physiological category as the autoimmune hypothesis is in (see chapter 11 on the History of Arthritis Research) ,

More research is urgently needed to explore the relation of potassium to rheumatoid arthritis. If you know a scientist able to perform such research, refer him to this article in the British Medical Journal [http://www.bmj.com/cgi/eletters/318/7190/1023].

Osteoarthritis can not be corrected using potassium, or at least using potassium alone [Jones].

CELL POTASSIUM CONTENT DURING RHEUMATOID ARTHRITIS

It has been determined by LaCelle that the whole body potassium is significantly lower in older arthritics. The body can sink to almost half of normal in some cases [LaCelle]. Sambrook, et al, also find potassium is low in early rheumatoid arthritis [Sambrook]. LaCelle's finding is very significant and has been confirmed by Nuki, et al [Nuki]. Even if one assumed that the rheumatoid arthritis caused the potassium content, rather than the other way around, it would be good common sense to bring such an important mineral up to normal in view of potassium's usual role in prevention of heart disease. If you decide to use supplements instead of food, be sure to read chapter 8 first. It is strange that this finding has not created more interest, as a diagnostic clue if nothing else. Even if scientists are not interested, there is nothing stopping you from at least getting all the potassium that was originally in your food. When 30 meq of potassium in a glucose solution was injected into old people for 2-3 hours it caused only one sixth the rise in electrolyte aldosterone steroid hormone that is responsible for stimulating potassium excretion as it did in 35 year old people [Saruta]. I suspect that this was because the cell content of those older people was very low in potassium, so after adding some potassium they would still be low. Red blood cell potassium averages higher in arthritics than normal. You can not take this as negative evidence because red blood cell potassium shows no correlation with plasma potassium [Ladefoged]. This may be an adaptation to avoid circulatory collapse during potassium losing diarrheas.

One can not draw a sure conclusion from low potassium serum from the blood content alone and it is dependent on the status of hydrogen ion and chloride. The reason is that plasma can have wide swings in content. However, 80% of people with rheumatic heart disease have low blood plasma content [Sokolov]. Even cell content is not certain proof all by itself. What is needed is a controlled experiment in which only potassium is varied. There never has been such an experiment for rheumatoid arthritis up until recently. Rastmanesh has performed a controlled, double blind, month long, clinical trial with significant rises in cortisol and declines in pain [Rastmanesh] (see further discussion below at the end). Placebo controls have been challenged recently, but they are in order for potassium experiments because the hormone most involved in potassium excretion, aldosterone, is much increased by fear and anxiety. However there has been an experiment performed by Schick on one of the arthritic diseases of the arteries called polyarteritis nodosa, which was indicative. Unfortunately cortisone was administrated at the same time so the experiment was flawed. However, everyone given 1.5 to 3 grams of potassium supplements per day had a complete healing of all arteries [Schick]. Potassium citrate was able to prevent arterial lesions in sodium chloride loaded hypertensive dahl rats without lowering the blood pressure. Potassium chloride had a somewhat lesser protective affect [Tobian]. I suspect that these affects on the blood vessels by potassium arises because a potassium deficiency inhibits cortisol production [Ueda] [Mikosha], which cortisol decline inhibits lysyl oxidase, the enzyme that cross links blood vessel connective tissue. This is probably the reason why low serum potassium is a risk factor in Kawasaki disease aneurysms [Koyanagi] and why a chief cause of death of rheumatoid arthritis patients is ruptured aneurysms [Matsuoka]. The rupture of aneurysms is no doubt accentuated by the high blood pressure that is associated with rheumatoid arthritis [Panoulas]. Vasculitis similar to polyarteritis nodosa is the most fatal of systemic complications [Hollingsworth]. Potassium chloride supplements prevent kidney damage in sodium loaded spontaneously hypertensive rats [Ellis]..There is also a single case history in which a subject was injected with various steroid hormones for a short time, each to determine their effect. The only consistent change during the course of the experiment was that his daily intake of potassium was raised to 3500 milligrams per day. His arthritic symptoms showed a consistent improvement throughout the course of the experiment even though some of the hormones used increase potassium excretion [Clark]. Now an unpublished experiment has been performed by Rudin on arthritics in which potassium supplements showed favorable results on eight patients [private communication]. In an experiment unrelated to rheumatoid arthritis, serum potassium was not improved with 1 gram of potassium per day unless magnesium was supplemented also. This was because magnesium is necessary in order to power the potassium pumps no doubt. Potassium can not be absorbed efficiently in the presence of a magnesium deficiency at least partly because the body cells can not absorb potassium Then [Ryan, p100]. Potassium can be impossible to absorb during a magnesium deficiency. Furthermore, a magnesium deficiency increases aldosterone secretion, which increases potassium excretion [http://www.lef. org/prod_hp/abstracts/php-ab236.html#3]. An experiment supplementing both would be in order in the future during arthritis in order to get crisper correlations.

Spironolactone has been found to improve juvenile arthritis and other types of rheumatoid arthritis [Bendtzen] Spironolactone is a substance that inhibits the action of aldosterone, which is the hormone that stimulates potassium excretion. This is a rather ridiculous way to get cell potassium up. Nutritious food is the preferred way.

Systemic lupus erythmatosis (SLE or lupus) has caused such extensive damage to kidney tubules that the patients had chronic high plasma potassium which was not responsive to aldosterone [De Pronzo]. Since Lupus patients have been shown to have visibly damaged tubules in 66% of patients examined, the investigators believe that this hyperkalemia is more common than realized. Since Lupus is listed as one of the arthritic diseases and has some similar symptoms, there may be a temptation to use supplements to heal it. Not only should this probably not be attempted, but also even foods high in potassium may be undesirable in the light of this report. Maybe some lupus victims' potassium intake must have a narrow safe range. Research to cast light on this would be highly desirable. Several circumstances have been found to act oppositely in arthritis caused by lupus such as pregnancy, estrogen, and schizophrenia [Mawson].

EVIDENCE

It is my contention that rheumatoid arthritis is essentially a chronic potassium deficiency, or more likely is greatly affected by one. Lending some circumstantial support to this proposal is that expression of voltage-gated K+ channels in mAb-defined T cell subsets from normal mice and mice with experimental autoimmune arthritis was studied with the patch-clamp whole-cell recording technique in combination with fluorescence microscopy. CD4+CD8- The cells from DBA/1 LacJ mice with type II collagen arthritis expressed low levels of type n K+ channels, and CD4-CD8+ T cells (cytotoxic) showed small numbers of type l or n' K+ channels, like their phenotypic counterparts in normal mice. CD4-CD8-Thy-1.2+ (double negative or DN) T cells from the diseased mice, however, displayed an abundance of type l K+ channels compared to DN T cells in normal mice. Furthermore, the aberrant expression of type l K+ channels correlated with the presence of active disease [Grissmer]. It may be that some genetic difference like sexual hormones, or differences in secretion of other hormones such as the glucocorticosteroid response modifying factors (GRMFs), or some other imbalance with other nutrients such as copper affect who, when, and how rheumatoid arthritis strikes. Obviously any disease or poison that interferes with retention of potassium would increase the chance of a deficiency developing. Considering that some of the symptoms of a deficiency take a long time to heal, it seems as if a deficiency should be avoided with almost the same urgency as a water deficiency (dehydration). Also, a deficiency of, say, 40 or 50 thousand milligrams would take a fairly long time to be completely corrected by food since getting more than 3500 milligrams per day from food is difficult and not all of it is retained. It would probably be measured in weeks at least. Potassium as potassium chloride would be much faster. In most cases, the worst reversible symptoms would probably disappear in a week or so if a thousand milligrams of potassium were added to each meal in that case. Potassium as the chloride raises blood pressure slightly. However, the differences are insignificant in humans [He]. Any slight differences may be because of difficulty in handling hydrogen ion (acid) in some forms of high blood pressure. Support is given to this possibility since sodium bicarbonate lowered blood pressure 5 mm of mercury while sodium chloride had no affect [Luft], possibly partly because sodium chloride was already high in their diet. Both sodium and chloride are necessary for pressure augmentation [Boegshold] perhaps operating through the sodium/potassium cell wall pumps, considering that a few essential hypertensive people have a genetic defect in those pumps [Garay]. This phenomenon may be involved with 18hydroxy-deoxycorticosterone steroid hormone (18OHDOC) because that hormone is raised in one of the forms of high blood pressure and that hormone is the hormone used by the body to increase acid excretion. Potassium is probably the main circumstance though, because vegetarians had consistently much lower blood pressure than non vegetarians in the same urban setting even though the sodium intake (and therefore chloride) of both groups was the same [Ophir]. See chapter 8 for more discussion of supplements..

Also limited experience makes me suspect that acids accentuate some types of headaches and potassium chloride should give the same effect as adding hydrochloric acid to a normal diet. If supplements are used, magnesium at least must be considered because magnesium is necessary for potassium absorbance. Also a vitamin B-1 deficiency (beriberi) becomes very dangerous for vitamin B-1 type of heart disease (wet heart disease of beri-beri) from potassium supplements [Folis] as discussed in chapter 3. This last situation could be involved for those who imbibe foods that contain sulfites because sulfites destroy vitamin B-1 in the intestines. The reverse would also be the case and so taking vitamin B-1 supplements should be dangerous for arthritics since heart disease is more common among rheumatoid arthritics than others, probably because of their low cell potassium. Osteoarthritis is probably the same as other healthy people in this regard. So unprocessed, nourishing food very high in not boiled vegetables is probably usually the best and safest way to get both potassium and vitamin B-1.

If "rheumatoid arthritis" or "potassium induced heart disease" are not words describing a potassium deficiency then what is the word equivalent to "beriberi" which describes a chronic potassium deficiency? Hypokalemia or hypopotassemia are not such words. They simply are words indicating a very low plasma content, with symptoms of lower T wave on the electrocardiogram, drowsiness, nausea, muscular weakness, low blood pressure, reduced digestive ability [Robinson], tachyarrhythmias, fibrillation, memory impairment, confusion, anorexia, constipation, lethargy, apathy, fatigue, depression, headache, irritability, and visual disturbance [Lindeman] (but for some reason hypokalemia induced by testosterone does not affect the electrocardiogram [Goldberger p113]). It would seem strange to have no word that describes the degenerative disease or diseases that accompany a chronic cellular potassium deficiency. I would suggest that we find one soon. Perhaps "cardiopotass" or "cardiokalium" would do for potassium deficiency caused heart disease.

CHAPTER 5
GOUT

SUMMARY

Causes of gout by lead and other poisons is presented. How to cure gout using potassium bicarbonate is shown, as well as orotate and coffee as ameliorators. Some of the history of gout is mentioned.

Gout is a disease in which sodium urate crystals are deposited in cartilage, especially in the feet. 90% of victims are men, perhaps because men are more likely to come in contact with lead (see below). The crystals are thought to be ingested by white blood cells and produce inflammation by rupture of the lysosome sacs and release of their contents [Turner]. Urate is the major end product of purine (nucleoproteins) degradation in higher primates in contrast to most other mammals because of the genetic silencing of hepatic oxidative enzyme uricase [http://en.wikipedia.org/wiki/Uric_acid]. The kidneys play the dominant role in urate excretion. The kidneys excrete 70% of the daily urate production and the intestines the remainder [Naohiko].

Lin has statistical evidence linking gout to lead poisoning [Lin 2002]. The lead poisoning makes the aldosterone system insensitive to potassium concentration and increases the potassium content of the blood plasma [Gonzalex]. The blood lead content is no indicator of toxicity and the status must be obtained with an EDTA mobilization test [Batuman]. Lead level in the body is significantly correlated with urate excretion and gout [Lin 2002]. Ethylenediaminetetraacetic acid chelator of lead has successfully increased uric acid excretion [Lin 2001]. Fluoride (now foolishly added to drinking water) has been suggested to increase lead intake. Other poisons than lead may move one a little closer to gout also, such as timalol (Blocadren) combined with hydrochlorothiazide and amiloride (a diuretic) [Greenly]. I also suspect that toluol or some other solvent in acrylic automobile enamel, which is actually a lacquer, may be able to trigger gout, from personal experience and I also suspect echinacea herb.

I have no information in the medical literature on any direct link between gout and a potassium deficiency. I have a strong suspicion that there is a link however. I have heard of a doctor who gave his patients potassium losing diuretics and thus triggered an attack of gout. By adding a potassium supplement he was able to remove the gout. Another doctor has used potassium supplements for his patients for years for the treatment of gout [private communication]. Gout can be triggered by the same agents that cause potassium losses such as fasting, surgery, and potassium losing diuretics [Rodman]. A potassium deficiency can increase urate levels in the blood [Davis] so there is a circumstantial connection. Urate kidney stones form during gout in 10-30% of cases [Colton]. Making the urine less acid (acidic (?))with potassium citrate or sodium bicarbonate is a current treatment for kidney stones [Shekarriz] [Rodman]. Potassium citrate has been successfully used to eliminate urate stones [http://www.nature.com/ki/journal/v30/n3/abs/ki1986201a.html]. I suspect that potassium bicarbonate or citrate would be preferable to potassium chloride for curing gout, but I have no other clinical evidence. I suspect this because uric acid is less soluble in acidic solution and potassium chloride added to a junk food diet should be equivalent to adding hydrochloric acid to a nutritious diet. I have removed gout symptoms over the course of several days by taking large potassium bicarbonate supplements of 1000 milligrams several times a day The initiating factor is probably most often lead poisoning though [Wright]. There is an association in people's minds between gout and rich foods and lifestyle, probably because people with gout have trouble excreting nitrogen in a soluble form and nitrogen is high in expensive meat, and perhaps also because wine bottles and plumbing contained lead in the distant past [http://www.doctoryourself.com/lead.html], Wine bottles and plumbing were mainly available to affluent people back then. It has been said that 10 generations of Roman aristocracy died out because of lead poisoning. It must have been a painful way to die because of the associated gout. Until such time as the matter is elucidated, it would be a good idea to stop eating lead, eat less proteins (especially purines), not allow any potassium to be lost from one's food, and take potassium bicarbonate supplements if you have gout. It has been suggested that maybe proteins from low fat dairy products may not exaggerate gout. Cherries have been shown to decrease urate in the urine of healthy women [Jacob], so they may have some therapeutic value. Some support to this possibility is that one half pound of cherries relieved the gout in 12 people [Blau]. It is possible that there is a substance in cherries that retards potassium excretion. There is some anecdotal evidence that celery and lettuce will relieve gout. If so, their high potassium content is probably what is involved. There is a discussion of current alternate treatment for gout online, which include black cherries [http://www. seekwellness.com/gout/what_is_gout.htm#alternative].

One would think that people with kidney failure, which causes potassium retention, would not have gout, but I know of no evidence for such a correlation. Uric acid itself is not a factor in heart disease because uric acid does not correlate with mortality from heart disease when damage to the heart and kidneys is taken into account [Lazzeri].

Orotic acid has been recommended for gout since it decreases uric acid. Orotic acid is Pyrimidinecarboxylic acid, also known as vitamin B13, Animal Galactose Factor, Oro, Orodin, Oropur, Orotonin, Oroturic, Orotyl, or whey factor. Vitamin B13 is not usually recognized as a vitamin. It is manufactured in the body by intestinal flora. It is normally used for a maximum of six days in Gout patients. Orotic acid is not necessarily always good in excess since it is said to bind zinc to a non-biologically active state and can damage the liver, but I would think that the 50 to 100 milligrams that has been recommended for normal supplementation should be safe, especially for a short time. Sources of oratate are whey, yogurt, beetroot, carrots, and jerusalem artichoke.

Drinking coffee but not tea has been found to lower uric acid in the serum so this effect is not likely to be from the caffeine [Kiyohara] or the potassium.

I suspect that none of the above when combined would have any significant bad health effects other than possibly the lead chelating chemicals, so it may be that we already have an affective cure for gout. It would be a good idea to find out for sure.

CHAPTER 6
DIABETES, TREATMENTS AND POSSIBLE CAUSES

SUMMARY

A brief history of diabetes is presented. There are some mitigating procedures you can adopt. Potassium is extremely important during diabetes and all aspects of too little and too much are discussed. Magnesium is also important and it is discussed. Vitamin B-3 may be able to reverse even type 1 diabetes. The nutrients taurine, inositol, alpha lipoic acid, acetyl L carnitine, and maybe flavinoids have advantageous affects on diabetes, Chile pepper is proposed as a possible cause of type 1 diabetes. A number of other causes of diabetes are discussed, including other poisons, Deficiencies of vitamin D, chromium, pyridoxine, vitamin B-6, zinc, copper, omega oils, iodide , and probiotics will make diabetes worse.

Diabetes can be seriously debilitating, initially leading to constant fatigue, somnolence and blurred vision, and if left untreated, progressing to eye deterioration, nerve deterioration, blindness, limb amputations, heart disease, diseases of the organs, hypertension, coma, and death. It costs 213-396 billion dollars worldwide with the country of Nauru spending 40% of the health care budget there on it. Diabetics in the USA lose $12,000 more than healthy people each year.

The brain does not need insulin to absorb glucose as do the other cells (except for the hunger center of the hypothalamus [Debons]), but it still can be affected by diabetes indirectly. The most noticeable symptom is insatiable thirst coupled with frequent urination. The body works overtime as it flushes glucose out, along with a loss of water, electrolytes and other minerals. Other symptoms include dizziness, tingling in feet and hands, thrush, genital itching, weight loss and extreme tiredness. If left to go its own course glucose cannot be used as a fuel, and so the body mobilizes its fat reserves as a source of energy. This is what causes rapid weight loss. The liver also converts fats to ketone bodies as an alternative fuel for the brain and other organs that are capable of using them. Ketone bodies are acidic, and in excess concentration cause ketoacidosis that can lead to coma.

Diabetes has been steadily rising since 1989 in the United States [http://www.cdc.gov/diabetes/statistics/prev/national/figbyage.htm]. Diabetes is the leading cause of new blindness in working-age adults, of new cases of end-stage renal disease and of non-traumatic lower leg amputations. In addition, cardiovascular complications are now the leading cause of diabetes-related morbidity and mortality, particularly among women and the elderly. In adult patients with diabetes, the risk of cardiovascular disease (CVD) is three-to-five fold greater than in the general population. Diabetes is the seventh leading cause of death in the United States and costs the American economy approximately $98 billion annually [http://diabetesmonitor.com/b307.htm]. It has been found that autoantibodies, including islet cell antibodies (ICA), glutamic acid decarboxylase antibodies (GADA), and antibodies directed against protein tyrosine phosphatase/IA2 (IA2-Ab), appear in the circulation years before clinical onset of diabetes and permit increasingly precise disease prediction [Gale].

I will attempt to explore the affect of insulin on other hormones, especially cortisol, to suggest that some poison in food may be causing diabetes, and to touch on some dietary considerations, especially potassium and copper.

Sugar diabetes, type 1, is caused by a destruction of the isles of Langerhan cells (beta cells) in the pancreas. These cells secrete insulin, a peptide or small chain amino acid hormone that regulates the transposition of glucose into the cells. In spite of years of experience in injecting insulin into the body to thwart this defect, people with diabetes have poor health. This poor health manifests itself as degeneration of the feet and eyes, among many other things.

One major problem which people with type 1 diabetes face is that the insulin is injected episodically in massive doses. Because insulin, as is the case with most peptide hormones, has a short half-life in the blood stream, measured in only a few minutes for insulin [Hoffman], insulin is cleared by the liver in about 15 minutes. The concentration in the body varies over wide extremes. The body has a way of varying the secretion of other hormones in an attempt to keep the most important parameters of physiology at a reasonably optimum level. However, compensating for insulin's variation can result in some disadvantageous compromises.

MITIGATING PROCEDURES

For instance, after large amounts of insulin enter the body, serum sugar content drops precipitously. Probably in an effort to correct this rather dangerous situation, there is a sudden upsurge in cortisol secretion [New England Journal of Medicine]. Cortisol gives effects which ramify throughout the body. The effect that the body is undoubtedly utilizing in this case, is the degradation of many proteins in order to produce glucose from them. The connective tissue is especially degraded [Houck], probably because this is the tissue that the body can most afford to lose short term. There is also a suggestion that insulin's indirect affect in increasing hydrogen ion or acidity (decreasing pH), because of potassium entering the cell with the glucose to form glycogen, could be an important part of health degradation [Moore 1986]. One way to avoid this would be by continuous infusion or by much more numerous injections of smaller doses with a high-pressure injector. It seems to me that it would also be helpful to eat glucose producing foods before the injection rather than after if both the above strategies are impractical in a particular case or time. Eating foods high in potassium should be advantageous also because one of the steroid hormones used to stimulate excretion of potassium, 11deoxycorticosterone (DOC), inhibits glycogen formation [Bartlett], so presumably potassium withdrawal into the cells would be more of a problem when that hormone declines. Blood glucose homeostasis requires that fasting concentrations lie between 35 and 58 millimoles per liter. This is termed the basal level (Waugh & Grant 459). Most health professionals agree that avoidance of high blood glucose concentrations is the number one priority for anyone suffering from diabetes, and, although it may not be number one, it is undoubtedly important. The way this is handled by diet is with complex carbohydrates called starch, which consist of long chains of glucose molecules and are created by plants. If eaten in the form that the plant created it, the plant tissues serve to delay the digestion (break down) of the carbohydrate. However, if the carbohydrate is processed by, for example, milling or grinding, it becomes more easily digested. If the carbohydrate is subjected to moist heat it is hydrolyzed, as in the baking and boiling process, and becomes gelatinized. (Garrow p65). In this form, it is readily converted to maltose by pancreatic amylase, which in turn is rapidly converted to glucose by the liver. Pritchford claims that a whole food diet with well chosen foods can eliminate the need for medicines in type 2 diabetes (formerly called non-insulin dependant diabetes or NIDDM) and external insulin in most people, even mitigating type I diabetes somewhat (Pitchford pp371-377). In my opinion, raw seeds such as oatmeal and wheat (wheat soaked in water) can be digested and taste at least as good as the slimy porridges and bland breads otherwise eaten. See this site for a defense of glycemic index, which term embodies the above concept [http://www.mendosa.com/wolever.htm]. Of course some foods such as potatoes and cabbage must or should be baked or cooked because they have mild poisons in them that are destroyed by heat. Eating diets high in dairy products, vegetables, fruits, and low in alcohol reduces the incidence of type 2 diabetes in Japanese men [http://jn.nutrition.org/cgi/content/abstract/136/5/1352]. However, it was undoubtedly primarily the vegetables and not the dairy products because it has been found that milk increases the insulin resistance of type two diabetes [http://care.diabetesjournals.org/cgi/content/full/28/10/2539], perhaps due to low copper of milk. So while milk may reduce the incidence of type 2 diabetes, it would seem that it increases the intensity of those who do get it. These strategies should be explored.

It has been suggested that the herbal sweetener, stevia, may have safe advantageous properties for diabetes. The advantages may be both for insulin production and for utilization [http://www.janethull.com/askdrhull/article.php?id=023] (I have no information on the safety of long term use. Because something is natural does not guarantee safety).

It has been discovered that pancreatic amyloid deposits of amylin are a hallmark of type 2 diabetes and considerable evidence indicates that amylin oligomers are cytotoxic (kill) to beta cells. Secoiridoid oleuropein aglycon, which is present in olive oil, consistently protected beta cells against toxicity of amylin [Rigacci].

Intake of 1 to 6 grams of cinnamon per day reduces serum glucose, triglyceride, LDL cholesterol, and total cholesterol in people with type 2 diabetes [Khan].

POTASSIUM

When glucose enters the cell, it takes potassium with it [Knochel 1997] to form glycogen, or animal starch. As a result, a dangerous, potentially lethal, low serum potassium can result. It is potentially lethal because the serum potassium must be kept at 4.8 milliequivalents per liter (187 milligrams per liter) [Lans] for nerve impulses to travel efficiently. For this reason, it is probably important for people with diabetes to eat foods adequate in potassium, including those foods eaten to provide immediate glucose. This would be especially important for those who still secrete insulin (type 2 diabetes) because people with a potassium deficiency secrete less insulin [Mondon] and potassium [Chattergee] as well as magnesium, vegetable oil, and calcium were inversely associated with type 2 diabetes for non-obese women [Colditz].

It is instructive to know what the possible causes of high blood potassium are. See chapter 7 for a discussion of high blood potassium. Most causes of high blood potassium are probably renal (kidney) failure. Diabetes causes over 30% of kidney failure for unknown reasons. In kidney failure during diabetes, potassium elevates after eating 100 grams of glucose, unlike normal people who show a slight decline [Knochel p447]. The slight decline in normal people is no doubt related to the fact that insulin, along with adrenaline stimulates the cell's potassium pump in muscles [Flatman]. I suspect that this in order to furnish potassium to form glycogen. I do not know what strategy diabetics with kidney failure should follow.

Glucose intolerance from low potassium develops exclusively associated with lower insulin secretion rather than the cellular response to insulin [Rowe] [Gardner]. The response time of insulin to glucose loading is also decreased in previously starved people by potassium supplements [Becker]. It could be an adaptation to avoid low plasma potassium resulting from the potassium entering into the cell in order to associate with glycogen that would otherwise occur. Low cell potassium can inhibit the insulin response independently of serum potassium [Spergel]. It is important to consistently get sufficient potassium in the diet because it takes a long time to rebuild low cell potassium and low cell potassium is very dangerous because of heart disease (Chapter 3). The cells have enormous amounts of total potassium normally, which is why it takes a long time to build it up if it becomes depleted.

Hyperglycemia can be managed by glucose-insulin-potassium (GIK) regimen [Das]. Use of GIK should keep in mind a new discovery that diabetics excrete vitamin B-1 at a much higher rate than other people, which leads to a vitamin B-1 deficiency [http://news.bbc.co.uk/1/hi/health/6935482.stm]. If potassium supplements are given during the wet heart disease of beriberi (thiamine or vitamin B-1 deficiency), the heart disease is made much worse [Mineno][Gould]. See chapter 3 for an extensive discussion of the interaction of vitamin B-1 with potassium during heart disease. Vitamin B-1 heart disease is impossible if potassium is also deficient [Folis]. Instead, a muscular atrophy similar to that from vitamin E deficiency appears [Hove] [Blahd]. During a vitamin B-1 deficiency the heart loses potassium [Mineno]. This may be why heart damage in beriberi or vitamin B-1 deficiency resembles that in a potassium deficiency. If you have heart disease it would be a good idea to try hard to find out which kind it is. If potassium is supplemented it would seem wise to supplement with vitamin B-1 as well or use foods high in it. Type 1 diabetics excrete vitamin B-1 four times more than normal people and type 2 diabetes three times, which leads to a vitamin B-1 content in plasma one fourth as high in diabetics. This is due to a malfunction of thiamine reabsorption in the proximal kidney tubules. It is probably the reason why high-dose thiamine and benfotiamine therapy increased transketolase expression in renal glomeruli, increased the conversion of triosephosphates to ribose-5-phosphate, and strongly inhibited the development of microalbuminuria. This was associated with decreased activation of protein kinase C and decreased protein glycation and oxidative stress, which are three major pathways of biochemical dysfunction in hyperglycemia [Babaei-Jadidi]. Erythrocyte vitamin B-1 was normal in diabetics, probably because there were increased thiamine transporters THTR-1 RFC-1 in the cell wall. Therefore erythrocyte thiamine can not be used to determine thiamine status [Thornalley]. If you decide to use potassium supplements instead of food, I recommend that you read Chapter 8 first.

Potassium in the blood was found to increase by use of sesame oil. In a study involving 40 hypertensive diabetic patients (22 male, 18 female) on medication (atenolol, a beta-blocker, and glibenclamide, a sulfonylurea anti-diabetic drug), using sesame oil in place of other cooking oils for a period of 45 days was found to bring about significant improvements. Subjects were given sesame oil (Idhayam Gingelly oil) and instructed to use it in place of their usual cooking oil for a period of 45 days. After 45 days of sesame oil use, both systolic and diastolic blood pressure reduced significantly. Furthermore, reductions were found in body weight, body mass index, girth of waist, girth of hip, waist/hip ratio, plasma glucose, HbA1c, TC, LDL-cholesterol, triglycerides, and plasma sodium levels, while plasma potassium levels increased. The activities of enzymic antioxidants and levels of nonenzymic antioxidants increased, while the levels of TBARS decreased. After 45 days of sesame oil use, the subjects were instructed to stop using sesame oil and instead cook with groundnut oil for 45 days. After this substitution, blood pressure was found to increase. The authors of this pilot study conclude that substitution of sesame oil as the sole edible oil has an additive affect in further lowering BP and plasma glucose in hypertensive diabetics [Sankar]. I do not know what it is in the sesame oil that does this.

The observations about potassium are reinforced circumstantially by a study that used a so called "vegan" diet with vegetables and legumes to cure type 2 diabetes, but no refined food, meat, or milk, which showed substantial improvement including much less loss of protein from the kidneys [http://www.pcrm.org/health/clinres/diabetes.html]. Milk removal can not be an important part of a reduction of incidence in type 2 diabetes because milk consumption in populations of men reduces incidence of type 2 diabetes [Choi and Walter], although, because it increases the severity of those who have type 2 diabetes, not drinking milk may be a good idea for them. Of course part of the above improvement of the vegan diet could have been increase of other nutrients, including vitamin C. It has been found that there was significantly less DNA damage when vitamin C was higher in the blood plasma in type 2 diabetes, that circumstance operative even in the presence of hyperglycemia [Choi and Benzie]. It is not necessary to give up meat, milk and eggs so far as potassium is concerned and they provide several essential nutrients that vegetables do not (see chapter 2).

MAGNESIUM

Calcium and magnesium, as well as potassium have been found to be inversely related to type 2 diabetes [Colditz]. Magnesium deficiency may be a common factor associated with insulin resistance and vascular disease [Nadler]. Low serum magnesium is a predictor of type 2 diabetes [Kao]. However, no correlation of type 2 diabetes with diet was observed [Kao]. So it could be that magnesium in most diets would be sufficient to prevent type 2 diabetes in the absence of some other factor, most likely a poison or a potassium deficiency. Potassium can not be absorbed efficiently in the presence of a magnesium deficiency and magnesium tends to be correlated with potassium intake. In a severe deficiency of magnesium, potassium can not be absorbed at all [http://www.mgwater.com/schroll.shtml]. So it is possible that the efficacy of magnesium is operating largely through its affect on potassium. Total body magnesium does not predict a deficiency, but blood serum must be low for that. If blood magnesium is 25% below normal, the enzymes depending on magnesium fail to operate adequately, including those responsible for its own absorption.

It has been proposed that magnesium and potassium supplementation would ameliorate vascular degeneration in at least a third of diabetics [Whang]. People with diabetes are prone to atherosclerosis, fatty degeneration of the liver and heart disease. People with diabetes have low magnesium tissue levels. They often develop eye problems (retinopathy), which are correlated with red blood cell and plasma magnesium [Durlach, a review]. People with diabetes who had the lowest magnesium levels had the most severe retinopathy (eye disease). The lower the magnesium content of their drinking water, the higher is the death rate of people with diabetes from cardiovascular disease. A larger percentage of magnesium is absorbed from water than is absorbed from food. In an American study the death rate due to diabetes was four times higher in areas with low magnesium as compared to areas with high levels of magnesium in the water. So magnesium supplements may be in order for diabetic people who eat junk food and maybe for everyone with diabetes of both types at times.

Magnesium (Mg) has been found to improve insulin sensitivity and metabolic control in type 2 diabetic patients [Rodriguez-Moran]. In non-insulin dependent diabetes (NIDDM or type 2) patients, daily magnesium administration, by restoring a more appropriate intracellular magnesium concentration, contributes to improved insulin-mediated glucose uptake. The benefits deriving from daily magnesium supplementation in type 2 patients are further supported by epidemiological studies showing that high daily magnesium intake are predictive of a lower incidence of type 2 diabetes (NIDDM) [Barbagallo].

It is possible to receive a lethal dose of magnesium just from gargling with Epsom salt (magnesium sulfate) [Gerard]. If this is so, this would be another argument for getting as much nourishment from food as possible and perhaps for not using excessive supplements of any nutrient interminably once body content is normal. Fung, et al, suggest that the reduction in risk for type 2 diabetes (NIDDM) from whole wheat is because of its magnesium content [Fung]. If so, green vegetables should be a good source because chlorophyll is made with magnesium

However magnesium chloride is said to be more advantageous than other forms for a wide variety of afflictions recognized as far back as 1914, including diabetes, asthma, bronchitis, pneumonia, emphysema, pharyngitis, tonsillitis, hoarseness, common cold, influenza, whooping cough, measles, rubella, mumps, scarlet fever; poisoning, gastro-enteritis, boils, abscesses, whitlow, infected wounds, and osteomyelitis. This is probably because absorbing as the chloride solves the hydrogen ion or acid/base problem. In more recent years Vergini and others have confirmed these earlier results and have added more diseases to the list of successful uses: acute asthma attacks, shock, tetanus, herpes zoster, acute and chronic conjunctivitis, optic neuritis, rheumatic diseases, many allergic diseases, chronic fatigue syndrome, and beneficial effects in cancer therapy [http://www.mgwater.com/vergini.shtml]. For a review of magnesium physiology and absorption, see Laires, et al [Laires]. It is very popular in Russia where they are amazed that it has not caught on in western medicine. Magnesium as the sulfate is probably not a desirable oral supplement since sulfate is an excretion product and the sulfate should have the same affect as adding sulfuric acid to a normal diet, whatever that is. Magnesium chloride could conceivably be in a similar position to some extent, especially during pain and probably if the kidneys are badly damaged. Also, it is the chloride in table salt that increases blood pressure, not the sodium [McCarty 2004][Boegshold], so magnesium as the chloride could turn out to be a disadvantageous form for people with high blood pressure.

One person reports getting red cell magnesium up to normal with magnesium orotate supplement and Epsom sulfate (magnesium as the chloride may be safer than the sulfate) foot baths every other day, along with choline citrate supplement in the hope the last helps with absorption. Magnesium as the orotate (Pyrimidinecarboxylic acid, also known as orotic acid or vitamin

B13, Animal Galactose Factor, Oro, Orodin, Oropur, Orotonin, Oroturic, Orotyl, or whey factor. B-13 is not really recognized as a vitamin because it is manufactured in the body by intestinal flora.) has been shown to be more readily absorbed than as the carbonate [Schlebusch]. Athletes had their swimming, cycling and running times decreased in the magnesium-orotate group compared with the controls and their insulin system markedly affected [Golf]. I suspect that this was primarily due to the orotate itself, because orotate is incorporated into RNA, enabled by biotin

[http://www.jbc.org/cgi/reprint/245/21/5600.pdf]. Biotin reduces blood glucose content in both type 1 diabetes [Reddi] and type 2 [McCarty 2007]. Orotic acid is not necessarily always good in excess since it is said to bind zinc to a non-biologically active state and can damage the liver. However, I would think that the 50 to 100 milligrams that has been recommended should be safe, but I have no sure information. Sources of orotate are whey, yogurt, beetroot, carrots, and Jerusalem artichoke, but not human milk. The importance of potassium is further reinforced by the fact that high serum concentrations of cortisol cause greater excretions of potassium [Barger]. If rheumatoid arthritis is involved, the situation is probably worse yet, because rheumatoid arthritics have a low whole body potassium content [LaCelle]. In addition, it may be that low insulin may cause greater excretion of potassium and magnesium because of affects on the energy furnished to their cell wall pumps. I have no information on this last. Disordered potassium metabolism that is expressed as hypokalemia (that is, a blood plasma potassium level below 3.5 mmol/L) can result in cardiac arrhythmias, muscle weakness, hypercalciuria, and glucose intolerance. Such disorders, which are correctable by potassium administration, can be induced by diuretics, chloride-depletion associated forms of metabolic alkalosis, and increased aldosterone production (Knochel, 1984). Low blood plasma reduces the capacity of the pancreas to secrete insulin and therefore is a recognized reversible factor in glucose intolerance (Helderman). There is some limited evidence that hypokalemia can also confer insulin resistance (Helderman), which is type 2 diabetes. A low potassium diet (580 milligrams per day), which did not induce frank hypokalemia, resulted in a decrease in plasma insulin concentration and a resistance to insulin action, which were reversed when dietary potassium was supplemented with 4800 milligrams per day (64 millimoles per day) of potassium chloride or about 2400 milligrams of potassium (Norbiato). Ideally potassium intake should total more than 3500 milligrams per day in my opinion and the FDA recommends 4,700. That last intake should be enough for almost all normal situations. Diuretic-induced-hypokalemia (low blood potassium) leads to insulin resistance (hyperglycemia and hyperinsulinemia) and glucose intolerance [Helderman]. Because moderate potassium deficiency and its adverse side effects can occur without hypokalemia, hypokalemia (low blood potassium) is not a sensitive indicator appropriate for use to establish adequacy. The first mild obvious adverse symptoms start to show up below about 4.4 milliequivalents per liter. Total body potassium is always depleted in diabetic ketoacidosis (DKA) but serum/plasma potassium may be low, normal or high [Yared]. Therefore, potassium must be corrected cautiously in that situation if supplements are used. In particular, it may yet prove to be mildly disadvantageous to use potassium chloride routinely. Use of this supplement should have the same affect as adding hydrochloric acid to a normal diet, whatever that is. In view of the wide spread use of low sodium table salt, this should be determined. Short term use is almost certainly safe, though, and it is the fastest way to get cell potassium raised.

There has been developed recently a test that uses electron bombardment of a single mouth mucous cell by electrons in order to generate distinctive x-rays [http://www.exatest.com/Research.htm]. It is said to determine other electrolytes inside the cell at the same time. This is very encouraging because previously, very expensive whole body scintillation counter machines were necessary to determine cell content.

The accepted view is that hyperglycemia (high blood sugar) results in glycosylation of protein, which is a cause of health problems during diabetes. However, it has been proposed that the acidity of cell fluid of people with diabetes, which shows up even when the blood serum is not abnormally acidic, may be a large part of those health problems [Moore 1991]. If this is so, using potassium supplements as the chloride or sulfate instead of as the bicarbonate may yet prove to be disadvantageous. Eating foods that have anions that can not be oxidized in the body, which many fruits and some vegetables no doubt have (but I have no information as to which ones), may be also disadvantageous. It is conceivable that this may even include vinegar and some citrus fruit, even though both the acetate and citrate are at least partly metabolized. In view of common use of these last foods, this matter should be explored.

You may see a site which discusses nutrients alleged to assist people with diabetes [http://www.doctoryourself.com/diabetes.html], but no discussion of potassium. People with type 2 diabetes should attempt to alleviate it as much as possible nutritionally. However, for those for whom nutrition does not take care of the problem completely, there are two compounds that show great promise if leptin deficient mouse experiments are an indication. They are 4-phenyl butyric acid (PBA) and an endogenous bile acid derivative ursodeoxycholic acid, the taurine conjugated derivative (TUDCA) [Ozcan]. These compounds have a good safety record and have been approved by the FDA for other diseases. Taurine amino acid itself seems to be advantageous and is easily obtainable. Taurine ameliorates kidney damage in general [Trachtman]. As much as 6 grams per day are said to be harmless [McCarty 2006, p67]. However taurine is not advantageous in protecting the kidneys from glomerular damage unless it is combined with N-acetyl-cysteine (NAC) in rats [Odetti].

I would suggest that a partial solution to the problem of poor potassium and magnesium nutrition would be to place a tax on all food that has had potassium or magnesium removed by food processors and use it to completely fund all Medicare and workman's compensation for injuries and disease that relate to diabetes, rheumatoid arthritis, heart disease, gout, high blood pressure, fibromyalgia, and chronic fatigue syndrome. This would also take the onerous tax burden now incurred for those diseases and place it on the shoulders of those who help cause the problem. To get such a law passed it will probably be necessary to convene a constitutional convention to reverse the Supreme Court ruling that corporations are individuals and can make unlimited political donations and ads because food processors will lobby vigorously against it and will bribe law makers.

It is said that some uncontrolled experiments have shown beneficial results using inositol (also called vitamin B-8) for diabetic neuropathy. Recommended dose is 500 milligrams twice daily. It is possible that this phenomena is related to inositol helping to power the potassium pumps [Bian] [Allard]. If so, getting enough potassium may be a better way and is no doubt at least partly necessary in this procedure. See this site for a discussion of nutrients which affect the potassium pumps, including inositol, especially as pertaining to pain during diabetes [http://www.aspartame.ca/page_a19a.html]. There is also evidence that alpha lipoic acid (ALA) will modulate insulin sensitivity in type 2 diabetes significantly [Ruus]. Acetyl-l-carnitine has shown promise to help prevent damage to the nerves of diabetics and reduce pain and enable nerve regeneration [Sima].

Life long supplementation with vitamin E has been proposed in order to minimize the oxidation of low density lipids and thus prevent or delay heart disease in type 1 diabetes [Engelen]. Also see this site [http://www.crnusa. org/vitaminEandhearthealth.html]. Of course, most of those supplements should not be necessary if wheat germ is eaten.

An experiment using cocoa significantly improved the cardiovascular function of ten people with type 2 diabetes. The researchers attributed this to flavinoids [Balzer].

It has been found that shields against electromagnetic radiation enable some people to have less severe symptoms of type 1 and 2 diabetes [Havas].

CHILI AS A POSSIBLE CAUSE OF TYPE 1 DIABETES

An interesting phenomenon associated with diabetes is that Hispanic people in Texas have three times the rate of diabetes as Anglicans. One in ten adult Hispanics have diabetes. The chance that this is a genetic defect by itself is extremely small. 62-94% of the time only one twin has diabetes, which all but rules out a genetic defect. Diabetes in previous years was invariably fatal, so there would be little chance of such a recessive gene remaining in the population in such large numbers. There is a chance that mitochondria genes are involved peripherally [Wallace], but it is highly unlikely that the ongoing type of mitochondria genetic damage implied with this could be dramatically different in the races in the absence of an environmental circumstance as well. There is little chance that a microorganism is involved directly since these people live in close association with each other. In any case, years of search have failed to show any pathogen. Recent research hints at a virus as part of the cause [von Harrath], but no definitive proof exists. A poison in the air seems unlikely since pure air blows off the Gulf most of the year. Besides, everyone is breathing the same air. The last circumstance is also true of water. This leaves food, the most important circumstance in our environment. There is a good chance that one of the foods which Hispanics eat more of than Anglicans has a poison in it which affects the isles of Langerhan disproportionately. All foods eaten in any quantity in greater amounts by Hispanics than others should be tested on primates in controlled experiments. I would be in favor of placing peppers high on the list, especially chili pepper [Weber 2008], since these come from a family of plants, Solanaceae, many of whose members have very vicious poisons. Chili peppers were domesticated in their Brazilian center of origination as long as 6000 years ago from a family of plants that probably originated in Bolivia [Perry]. It has been found that a substance in peppers known as capsaicin (8-methyl-N-vanillyl-6-nonenamide), along with a related compound (resiniferatoxin) placed on human skin cancer cells kills them [JNCI], so chili is a good candidate. Also capsaicin is mutagenic (causes genetic defects) [Nagabhushan]. A receptor, vanilloid receptor subtype 1 (VR1), forms a nonselective cation channel in the plasma membrane that mediates some of the effects of capsaicin and its analogues, which are named vanilloids. This is thought to be the mechanism for capsaicin's use to inhibit pain [Suth]. Chili is especially likely because capsaicin placed on the nerves surrounding the insulin cells in mice kills the nerves. Then, after the researchers injected the neuropeptide "substance P" normally deficient in the nerve cells in the pancreases of diabetic mice, the diabetes instantly cleared up and remained that way after one injection [http://www.canada.com/nationalpost/news/story.html?id=a042812e-492c-4f07-8245-8a598ab5d1bf&k=63970&p=2].

It is possible that preliminary evidence could be obtained by immersing isles of langerhan cell cultures in extracts of these foods. If any are found to be poisonous, perhaps the situation could be resolved by breeding the poison out of the edible parts. That chili could be involved is hinted at by virtue of the fact that insulin secretion is inhibited after a meal high in sugar is eaten with chili [Ahuja]. It is possible that chili acts in synergism (reinforce each other) with a copper deficiency since adequate copper prevents diabetes in ATZ poisoned mice [Sitasawad]. Capsaicin has been proposed for weight reduction, pain inhibition, and other purposes [http://naturalfoodsmerchandiser.com/tabid/66/itemid/3096/Spicing-up-health-with-capsaicin.aspx]. Before any of this is attempted, there should be long term experiments involving chili in conjunction with a copper deficiency with regard to diabetes. It is a very bad idea to use a medicine first and experiment with it afterwards.

Deborah Cavel-Greant [private communication] has pointed out that Hispanics have considerable Indian genes and that Indian tribes from Mexico to the Arctic have high rates of diabetes. She points out that her Tuscarora people of the Cree are plagued by diabetes and do not eat chili much. So, if they do not eat peppers much, and peppers are involved, something else may be also, or that Indians are more susceptible to chili than others. It is possible that there is a genetic component because diabetics have skin nerve regeneration more inhibited by capsaicin than non-diabetics [Polydekis]. A survey should be performed to determine this. The Pima Indians have a higher diabetes rate than white people living nearby and they have a much higher chili consumption [Reid]. Pima Indians in Mexico have very low rates, but I do not know their chili intake. It is conceivable that marginal diabetes may have added an additional problem to the problem of poor resistance to introduced disease in explaining why the South and Central American Indians collapsed so quickly before the advance of the Europeans.

A worldwide study of the incidence of juvenile diabetes showed variations of 350 fold between regions. There were no correlations with ethnicity or races or climate. So some kind of poison still seems to be all that is left. If so, it would be very desirable to find out what it is. If there is a poison in food, it should be easy to determine what it is.

OTHER POSSIBLE CAUSES

Chili can not be the only diabetes poison if it is a poison, for a study found a 47 percent increase in diabetes among veterans with the highest levels of dioxin in their bloodstream. Dioxin is the compound in Agent Orange linked to bad health effects in laboratory animals. The result is based on 1997 physical examinations of 1,000 Air Force veterans who were exposed to

Agent Orange during the nine years that it was used as a defoliant and crop killer in Vietnam.

It has been found that bafilomycin, a toxin found in some bacteria called streptomyces that infect vegetables such as potatoes, sugar beets, turnips and radishes, may predispose babies of mothers who eat such food to diabetes. Pregnant mice that ate tiny amounts of the toxin, which cannot be destroyed through cooking, were far more likely to have babies that later developed type 1 diabetes. The evidence is backed up by a high rate of diabetes in Finland and Sardinia, where root crops are eaten in large amounts.

A large number of other poisons added to food have been proposed to increase the risk of diabetes. They include arsenic, alloxan, aspartame, MSG, benzene, bisphenol A in container plastic, pthalates, and pentachlorophenol (PCP) [http://www.naturalnews.com/023701.html]. Lectins, plant proteins which bind certain carbohydrates, have been proposed as making certain cells susceptible to autoimmune destruction [http://bmj.com/cgi/content/full/318/7190/1023].

Another poison which may yet be shown to predispose to diabetes is the drug, olanzapine (trade name Zyprexa), belonging to a relatively new family of medications called atypical antipsychotics, which are used to treat schizophrenia, paranoia and manic-depressive disorders. Other drugs in this class include clozapine, risperidone, quetiapine and ziprasidone. The researchers found metabolic abnormalities ranging from mild blood sugar problems to diabetic ketoacidosis and coma in patients who had been prescribed olanzapine, most of whom were otherwise not known to be diabetic [http://www.eurekalert.org/pub_releases/2002-07/dumc-rwa062802.php]. Diabetic ketoacidosis (DKA) is a serious condition in which a person experiences an extreme rise in blood glucose level coupled with a severe lack of insulin, which results in symptoms such as nausea, vomiting, stomach pain and rapid breathing. Untreated, DKA can lead to coma and even death.

Aspartame, a zero calorie sweetener added to food, has been found to accentuate diabetes. It has been proposed that aspartame will damage the hypothalamus, which part of the brain controls steroids and seems to be defective in chronic fatigue syndrome (CFS, ME, or CFIDS). Aspartame degrades to the very poisonous methyl alcohol (methanol), poisonous because it can become formaldehyde. Aspartame is suspected to cause blindness, systemic lupus, maybe heart disease [Lutsey], and cancer [Soffritti] among other things, and mimics multiple sclerosis in some people. One of my respondents proposes that the chemical structure mimics 'real' phenylalanine, and is selectively/preferentially able to cross the blood-brain barrier into the brain, where it locks into place, preventing the 'real' chemical from getting to where it's supposed to go. See this site for Dr. Christine Lydon's discussion of some of its affects and history of the politics of getting it declared safe [http://www.aspartamekills.com/lydon.htm]. If you would like to write a letter to your state or federal legislator, you can see an elaborate letter for that here [http://www.mpwhi.com/project_recall_aspartame.htm]. It is a good idea not to eat or drink anything laced with aspartame. If you have been eating aspartame there is a web site that suggests some ways of detoxifying it [http://www.wnho.net/wtdaspartame.htm]. If you use the vitamin B-1 as they suggest, be absolutely certain that your potassium is adequate or you could trigger a heart attack (see chapter 3).

Also, it has been found recently that persistent organic pesticides (POPs) absorbed by eating fish are associated with type 2 diabetes [Lee 2007]. The researchers entertained the possibility that type 2 diabetes make people absorb persistent organic pesticides more readily than others, rather than the other way around. However, they think this is unlikely. They find that these poisons are synergistic with obesity. This may explain why obese people seem to be more prone to type 2 diabetes. However, it is not likely obesity itself that makes people prone, but rather a sedentary life style, a life style that causes both the obesity and poor health [Charansonney].

It has been shown that degradation products from over cooked foods make mice prone to diabetes more susceptible after eating foods high in those products [Zheng].

NUTRIENTS

Large doses of vitamin B3 (nicotinamide, niacinamide, or niacin) prevents onset of type 1 insulin dependent diabetes [Kolb]. They believe that cell death pathways are modified through affects on poly (ADP-ribose) polymerase (PARP), and to a lesser extent (mono) ADP-ribosyl transferases (ADPRTs). 26 milligrams per kilogram of body weight were just as affective as 50 [Visalli]. Children with antibodies treated with vitamin B-3 (niacin) had less than half the onset of diabetes incidence in a 7 year time span as the general population and even lower incidence relative to those with antibodies as above, but no vitamin B-3 [Elliot 1996] [Mandrup]. The mechanism of action appeared to the investigators to be (a) inhibition of macrophage and interleukin-1-mediated beta cell damage and (b) inhibition of nitric oxide production. The anti-oxidant role of B-3 may also be involved [Andersen], although I doubt it myself. This would seem to indicate that a vitamin B-3 deficiency should be avoided, and in particular, to eat NO refined flour and to eat little corn. Vitamin B-3 deficiency causes pellagra disease. Niacin itself is not toxic, but the chemicals converted by niacin are toxic to the skin and liver in overdose, and high doses of niacin should only be reached with gradual increase.

Petrie recommends no more than 250 milligrams per day for adults [private communication see http://tompetrie.net/]. He believes that type 1 diabetes can be cured if it is caught before all the isles of Langerhan cells have died (newly diagnosed) using niacinamide or vitamin B-3, but not the nicotinic acid form. He is backed up by a study of newly diagnosed type 1 diabetes in children in which three patients out of seven were in clinical remission after one year, but none in the placebo group [Vague]. This procedure was first proposed by Lazerow in 1950 [Lazarow].

Of course, nutritional deficiencies or imbalances can not be ruled out as contributory factors yet and may yet prove to partly treat diabetes. There have been studies that indicate that vitamin D supplemented in the first year of life reduces diabetes in later years. Children treated with 2,000 IU daily of vitamin D from their first birthday onward had an 80% decreased risk of developing type 1 diabetes throughout the next 20 years [Hypponen], so I suspect that 5 times that amount would be safe for adults. People getting no sunlight should supplement with at least 1,000 IU of vitamin D, which is 5 times the usually recommended amount [Glerup]. The majority of normal people are too low in vitamin D also. Studies in the past establishing normal levels were based on the general population who are marginally deficient. They should have been based on levels in life guards. Recent studies reveal that current dietary recommendations for adults are not sufficient to maintain circulating 25(OH)D levels at or above 80 nmol or 32 µg/L, especially in pregnancy and lactation [Hollis]. Since naked Africans receive 10,000 IU, Vieth suggests that concerns of toxicity are inappropriate [Vieth]. A wide margin of safety above current intakes has been established [Kimball]. Masterjohn proposes that vitamin D toxicity, when much too much is taken, is from a concurrent vitamin K and a vitamin A deficit [Masterjohn]. An additional advantage is that apparently epidemiological studies and circumstantial evidence show lower rates of multiple sclerosis, hypertension, osteoarthritis, and colorectal, prostate [Chan], inflammation, influenza, tuberculosis, breast cancer, and ovarian cancer when vitamin D is adequate [Tavera-Mendoza]. Some of these effects may be because of more efficient absorption of magnesium and calcium as enabled by vitamin D [Ritchie].

We are now able to better identify sufficient circulating 25(OH)D levels through the use of specific biomarkers that appropriately increase or decrease with changes in 25(OH)D levels. These include intact parathyroid hormone, calcium absorption, and bone mineral density. Using these functional indicators, several studies have more accurately defined vitamin D deficiency as circulating levels of 25(OH)D lower than 80 nmol or 32 µg/Liter. Recent studies reveal that current dietary recommendations for adults are not sufficient to maintain circulating 25(OH)D levels at or above this level, especially in pregnancy and lactation [Hollis].

Lack of sufficient exercise is already known to contribute to diabetes. You would think that exercise immediately after a meal would be most advantageous, in order to help mitigate the surge in blood sugar then, but I know of no clinical evidence. Being overweight or obese has been statistically linked to type 2 diabetes. I consider it unlikely that fat or fat cells themselves have a significant affect on diabetes, and fat as a cause has recently been discredited [Gibbs]. In any case, fasting should not be prolonged because muscle wasting is dangerous and weight reduction is not a factor in amelioration of rheumatoid arthritis, at least, from vegetarian diets. However, both overweight and diabetes linked to a third factor, such as not enough exercise or poor nutrition, is quite possible. Also, extra fat may be soaking up the fat soluble vitamin D, E, or A. It has been found that DHEA hormone supplements significantly decrease abdominal fat and insulin action in elderly people [Villereal]. It also has been shown that DHEA increases insulin sensitivity in type 2 diabetes [Dhatariya]. It would be advantageous to determine the mechanism. It would be a good idea to wait until long term experiments demonstrate that this is safe for sure. Other adrenal steroids have a dubious safety history.

Deficiencies of the nutrients chromium, magnesium, potassium, and pyridoxine (similar to vitamin B-6) are said to make worse hyperglycemia during pregnancy as discussed in the following abstract: "There is an increased requirement for nutrients in normal pregnancy, not only due to increased demand, but also increased loss. There is also an increased insulin-resistant state during pregnancy mediated by the placental anti-insulin hormones estrogen, progesterone, human somatomammotropin, the pituitary hormone prolactin, and the adrenal hormone, cortisol. If the maternal pancreas cannot increase production of insulin to sustain normal glycemia (sugar status) despite these anti-insulin hormones, gestational diabetes occurs. Gestational diabetes is associated with excessive nutrient losses due to glycosuria. Specific nutrient deficiencies of chromium, magnesium, potassium and pyridoxine may increase the tendency towards hyperglycemia in gestational diabetic women because each of these four deficiencies causes impairment of pancreatic insulin production. This review describes the pathophysiology of the hyperglycemia and the nutrient loss in gestational diabetes and further postulates the mechanism whereby vitamin/mineral supplementation may be useful to prevent or ameliorate pregnancy-related glucose intolerance" [Jovanovic-Peterson].

Vitamin B-6 supplementation has been found to reduce nerve damage in diabetics [Jain]. In cases of juvenile diabetes, there were lower than normal levels of reduced glutathione, ceruloplasmin oxidase activity, zinc, copper and sodium, while the other elements show no significant changes [Awadallah]. Zinc and arachidonic acid were found to lower glucose via improvement in insulin sensitivity in genetically diabetic rats [Song]. This may be because insulin requires zinc [Pfeiffer, p143]. Omega 3 and omega 6 vegetable oils have been found to protect against chemically induced diabetes [Suresh], so it could be that our current foolish custom of hydrogenating vegetable oils may be predisposing us to diabetes, at least type 2.

Because the amino acid, taurine, is thought to be advantageous for people with diabetes, magnesium taurate may be the best supplement to take [McCarty 2006]. Taurine supplements have been found to give some protection to the retinas of diabetic rats [DiLeo 2000, & 2003]. As mentioned in chapter 3, taurine (2-aminoethanesulfonic acid) is an acidic amino acid sulfonated rather than carboxylated, which is found in high abundance in the tissues of many animals, especially sea animals. Taurine is also found in plants, fungi, and some bacterial species, but in far less abundance. It is an amine with a sulfonic acid functional group, but it is not an amino acid in the biological sense, not being one of the twenty protein-forming compounds encoded by the universal genetic code. Small polypeptides have been identified as containing taurine, but to date there has been no report of a transfer RNA that is specifically charged with taurine [from Wikipedia]. It is essential to babies.

There is strong evidence that taurine could have beneficial affects on type 1 diabetes, and could reduce organ peroxidation and plasma lipids. The retina, lens, and nerves respond better to taurine than other organs [Franconi]. Taurine has been used for high blood pressure [Fujita], migraine headache (I suspect that less than 1000 milligrams of taurine can remove the headache caused by allergy to peanuts and some spices from personal experience), high cholesterol, epilepsy, macular degeneration [Bian] [Allard], Alzheimer's disease, liver disorders, alcoholism, cystic fibrosis, and depression. Keep in mind that some people may have a genetic defect that limits the amount of taurine tolerated and that adequate molybdenum may be desirable. Taurine may make a copper deficiency worse, based on a single case history [Brien Quirk, private communication]. This may be because taurine may be mobilizing copper and zinc into the plasma [Li]. So if you should decide to take taurine, make sure your copper intake is more than adequate, as well as possibly your zinc.

Experiments have indicated that acetyl-l-carnitine amino acid may reduce pain during diabetes, diabetic neuropathy, and maybe help in nerve regeneration and insulin resistance. It has shown safe advantageous affects on numerous diseases that are involved with the nervous system such as attention deficit hyperactivity disorder, Alzheimer's disease, chronic fatigue syndrome, multiple sclerosis [http://www.raysahelian.com/acetylcarnitine.html],

Copper depletion doubled glucose in blood of diabetic rats fed glucose, 50% higher for sucrose [Cohen]. There must be a couple of copper catalyzed enzymes somewhere in the processes, therefore. One investigator has suggested that buildup of copper in the kidneys of people with diabetes is responsible for the kidney damage which sometimes appears in people with diabetes (based on rats) [Gassman]. People with diabetes probably absorb copper two times more readily than normal people [Craft]. This may be the reason why diabetics have a reduced chance of getting an aortic aneurysm [Blanchard], due to copper catalyzed lysil oxidase cross linking of elastin in blood vessels. Therefore people with diabetes may have a narrow safe range of intake. It would be desirable to find out. It is possible that this is an adaptation evolved to help forestall a synergism of copper deficiency with a poison that causes diabetes. The pancreas can be irreversibly destroyed by a copper deficiency in rats inside a few months, but the isles of Langerhan are not affected [Smith] [Fell]. Even so, there is a somewhat negative correlation between copper in drinking water and the onset of juvenile diabetes [Zhao]. In cases of juvenile diabetes, there were lower than normal levels of reduced glutathione, ceruloplasmin oxidase activity, zinc, copper and sodium, while the other elements show no significant changes [Awadallah]. So it is possible that people with partial destruction of their beta cells could cut back on their medication with proper nutrition. As already mentioned in conjunction with chili, it is possible that adequate copper could help prevent insulin dependant diabetes since it does so for ATZ poisoned mice [Sitasawad] and copper in drinking water has a somewhat protective affect [Zhao]. It could be that copper produces its effects through super oxidase dismutase because it has been shown that the antioxidant metalloporphyrin-based superoxide dismutase (SOD) can prevent or delay the onset of the so called autoimmune cascade in diabetes, using mice as subjects. [Haskins].

Once insulin dependant diabetes sets in, handling copper may be a problem and may be part of the difficulty with poor health afflicting people with diabetes. It has been found that taking vitamin C supplements increases mortality from cardiovascular disease in diabetic post menopause women [Lee 2004]. This may be because of the fact that vitamin C increases the need for copper. Shellfish and liver are the richest food sources of copper, with leafy vegetables fairly high.

Houstis thinks that reactive oxygen species (ROS) cause type 2 diabetes. ROS are radical forms of oxygen that arise as by-products of mitochondrial respiration and enzymatic oxidases spurred on by TNF and dexamethasone (an analog of cortisol) [Houstis]. If so, this would be additional circumstantial evidence that copper is involved in type 2 diabetes, since it is copper catalyzed enzymes that remove ROS. Epidemiological evidence should be obtained to see if there is a correlation with aneurysms, hemorrhoids, herniated discs and other copper deficiency caused diseases.

Another nutrient which is probably helpful in type 2 diabetes is chromium. It must be in the trivalent form, in which form it is very safe [http://www. healingwithnutrition.com/mineral.htm]. Chromium picolinate will mute some of the affect that smoking has on insulin resistance [McCarty 2005]. There is considerable evidence that chromium is advantageous for type 2 diabetes. I have heard of a single case in which taurine chromium supplements considerably improved tinnitus ringing of the ears, which is often associated with type 2 diabetes. The Food and Nutrition Board of the National Research Council has recommended a "safe and adequate" range for dietary chromium of 50 to 200 mcg per day. Food intake analyses suggest that, on average, Americans consume below the adequate level. For example, one analysis of 22 diets designed to be well balanced showed a range of daily intakes from 8.4 to 23.7 mcg per 1,000 calories (mean 13.4 mcg) [http://www.newhope. com/nutritionsciencenews/NSN_backs/Feb_99/chromium.cfm] [Anderson 1992]. The signs and symptoms of chromium deficiency in mammals include impaired glucose tolerance, elevated circulating insulin concentration, glycosuria, fasting hyperglycemia, impaired growth, hypoglycemia (why it should cause both hypo- and hyper- I do not know), elevated circulating cholesterol and triglyceride concentrations, neuropathy, decreased insulin binding, decreased insulin receptor number and impaired humoral immune response. A junk food diet low in meat is probably the most likely way to be afflicted with a chromium deficiency. 1000 mcg of chromium picolinate per day was necessary to see the full range of body biochemical benefits in China [Anderson 1997a]. Chromium with a valence of three is not toxic in large amounts probably because chromium is absorbed less from high concentration. Chromium chloride and chromium picolinate have been fed to rats at thousands of times the National Research Council's upper limit (on a body-weight basis) with no evidence of toxicity [Anderson 1997b]. Other valence states of chromium ARE toxic though.

Fructose high in the diet will enhance insulin resistance [Elliot 2002]. This may be because of the adverse affect that fructose has on a copper deficiency.

Inositol is thought to increase sensitivity to insulin [Lamer], perhaps because of inositol's requirement for the electrolyte cell wall electrolyte pumps. It has been discovered that two anthocyanins, which are colored pigments in foods, cyanidin-3-glucoside and delphinidin-3-glucoside, stimulate insulin production [Jayaprakasam]. This may prove to be useful in type 2 diabetes.

There is always an element of risk in medicines that affect body functions, however. So more long term experience would be desirable before making extensive use of this.

Iodide reduces the amount of insulin necessary during type 1 and Type 2 diabetes. Iodide also can get rid of cysts in the ovaries, depression, cold extremities, night time leg cramps, and reduces the occurrence of breast cancer, stomach cancer, esophageal cancer, ovarian cancer and endometrial cancer. Iodide has been proposed to augment the immune system. It has also been proposed to mitigate the poisonous effects of bromide as well as the bad effects of fluoride currently foolishly added to more than half the drinking water in the USA.

Probiotics have been found to be advantageaos in preventing diabetes [Latinen][Yadev 2007][Yadev 2008]. A probiotic can be defined as a preparation of, or a product containing, viable, defined micro-organisms in sufficient numbers, which alter the microbiota by implantation or colonization in a compartment of the host and by that produce beneficial health effects in the host. Probiotic preparations and products most commonly contain strains of lactobacilli, bifidobacteria or saccharomyces, or mixtures of these strains. Probiotics for children during the first 6 months of their life reduces the antibodies that correlate with future risk of diabetes to almost zero [Lungberg]. Probiotics during pregnancy markedly reduced gestational diabetes [Luoto]. If so, I do not know the mechanism.

Using insulin to alleviate diabetes is a marvelous advance, but there is no excellent substitute for preventing the disease in the first place, and research should be directed to ruling out possible causal and contributing factors in our environment, especially foods. It is possible that, if all the poisons that are discovered affecting diabetes are removed and all of our food becomes nutritious by virtue of food processors not degrading it, diabetes might subside to a low incidence. Use of refined flour and sugar is without a doubt especially damaging in regard to nutritional deficiencies. White sugar has zero value. In addition, mental state is fairly important and there is evidence that blood sugar after meals is improved by laughter during meals.

At the very least, the known poisonous causes of diabetes in foods should be taxed and the revenues used to completely fund diabetes treatments and devices. That would be the most just and effective way.

You can see the web site of a diabetes foundation here [http://islet.org]. You can see some proposed theories regarding type 2 diabetes at this site [http://www.healingmatters.com/diabetes.htm]. There has been an experiment performed that transformed body cells into insulin secreting cells in mice [Zhou]. So there is hope of a cure in the future. An encouraging development for type I diabetes is the discovery that implanting the gene for cdk-6 in the kidneys of mice caused them to start to produce insulin [http://www.worldhealth.net/news/beta_cell_discovery_offers_hope_of_new_t]. It is possible that some day it will be possible to cure type 1 diabetes. I sure hope so.

SOME TERMS USED IN DIAGNOSING DIABETES

BG = Serum blood glucose concentration (90 is normal; above 140 is abnormal.) 400 is sufficient to be admitted to hospital. HbA1C - Haemaglobin Adult division 1c measures glycosylation of haemaglobin. Haemaglobin is recycled every 90-120 days so this is an indicator of excess serum glucose over that period. Below 5.5% is normal. Diabetic target range is 6.5% -7.5%, over that spells increased risk of heart disease, myopathy, amputations, blindness and death.

CHAPTER 7
HIGH BLOOD POTASSIUM OR HYPERKALEMIA

SUMMARY

High blood potassium (metabolic shock) can be caused by injury. The usual cause is kidney failure from diabetes, lupus erythmatosis, plaque build up, poisons (such as fluoride), or medicines. Prostate blockage from oil hydrogenation or a zinc deficiency can also cause high blood potassium. There are corrective procedures such as avoiding dehydration, eating sodium bicarbonate, eating less meat, drinking no wine, possibly using no glucosamine, eating no acidic foods, of course using no potassium supplements, making use of enemas and sweating, and hyperventilating.

Some people are afflicted with high potassium in their blood (metabolic shock or hyperkalemia). Even a fairly small consistent rise in serum or plasma potassium of 0.5 milliequivalents (meq) or so over the norm, which is 4.8 [Scribner], is cause for some concern, because a healthy body is capable of a rather precise regulation of potassium, and a considerable portion of the kidney (renal) function must be gone before symptoms start to show. In my opinion the potassium must rise 1.0 meq/liter or so before one would start to use the word alarm. The electrocardiogram changes at 6.5 meq [Seekles]. I believe the dangerous symptoms of metabolic shock start to materialize after about 7.0 meq. I believe death is possible in the vicinity of 8.0 meq at which point the first clinical symptoms of heart failure appear [Seekles] and that life is impossible beyond 10.0 meq or so. Very high potassium that

67

gives very noticeable symptoms is a MEDICAL EMERGENCY AND A HOSPITAL SHOULD BE SOUGHT. Only 2 or 3 decades ago potassium was not even listed in the index of books devoted to discussing metabolic shock, even though metabolic shock IS high blood potassium. It was another manifestation of the cavalier attitude of most medical professionals toward potassium then and to a considerable extent now. Potassium supplements were referred to by such euphemisms as "pharmaceuticals", "salt substitutes", "polarizing solutions", "GIK", and "ORT salts". It is so even today to some extent.

Before assuming that your potassium is too high, be sure that the analysis of blood is of plasma and not of serum since serum can give inaccurately high readings. Analysis of serum within one half hour would prevent the disparity [Bellevue]. This inaccuracy results when blood stands at low temperatures and potassium can leak from the cells and also there can be cell losses if the blood is handled roughly. Even without poor technique serum potassium will be higher than plasma by 0.2 meq/liter in normal subjects [Ifudu]. Even with careful determination plasma potassium can be anomalously high because of potassium losses from platelets during rheumatoid arthritis. A difference of 0.4 meq/liter can occur when platelets release potassium. [Ifudu]. If there is an inappropriate high reading there can be a degrading of health from the treatment itself as well as sometimes high, unnecessary expense. Electrocardiogram readings (ECG) can act as a check on serum analysis in the case of readings above 6.5 or so and effects in the heart are the most important manifestations anyway. As levels increase, the first ECG change is tall peaked T waves. The QT interval is normal or diminished. As potassium levels continue to rise, the PR interval becomes prolonged, and then the P wave amplitude decreases. The QRS complex widens into a sine wave pattern, with subsequent cardiac arrest.

There are things one can do to ameliorate high blood potassium temporarily at home, and I will propose some possible strategies. However, high blood potassium is a symptom of a rather serious underlying problem and you should contact a medical professional and make a great effort to find out what the problem is and correct it if at all possible. You may see mention of the symptoms of too high a blood potassium in [Recheigl]. Some symptoms are said to be irregular or fast heartbeat, paralysis of limbs, drop in blood pressure, convulsions, coma, cardiac arrest, black or bloody stool, diarrhea, confusion, breathing difficulty, vomiting, extreme fatigue, nausea, numbness, tingling hands and feet, and breathing difficult. The two most likely causes of a chronic situation are damaged kidneys or a hormone disruption. People tend to get despondent at such times, and not completely without reason. However, if the underlying cause is removed, and you then eat, drink, or breath (translate; smoke) no poison and receive all the nutrients originally in your food including most of a small amount of protein from high quality sources such as meat, eggs, and milk and no overwhelming amounts of any, say sodium, chloride, zinc, vitamin B-1, or phosphate (of soft drinks) and get plenty of exercise, it is my belief that there is a good chance that adequate healing will usually take place if the damage has not been overwhelming. One contraindication to the value of excessive exercise is probably chronic fatigue syndrome or also called CFS, ME or CFIDS. The body has considerable power to repair itself for most tissue, although I am not certain of the kidney's ability to do so. If there has been extensive damage to the kidneys it probably will not be possible to return completely back to normal especially in people past 15 years of age or so, but this need not be cause for despair because a healthy pair of kidneys has much more capacity than they need to just maintain normal life. Healthy kidneys are said to be able to unload 26,000 mg of potassium in a day if necessary [Peterson]. So losing some capacity is not necessarily ruinous. I could be mistaken in this, but if it were me, I would not give up trying, even if I was on a dialysis machine. Keep in mind that people beyond 50 or 60 usually heal up slowly though, and much more than a year may be necessary if it is possible. In the rare cases when a genetic defect is involved the underlying problem may be intractable. However some reasonable changes in lifestyle may nevertheless ameliorate even those situations.

CAUSES OF HIGH BLOOD POTASSIUM

It is instructive to know what the possible causes of high blood potassium are. Most of them are probably renal (kidney) failure. Diabetes causes over 30% of kidney failure for unknown reasons (see chapter 6). About 30% are related to hypertension (but not necessarily caused by it), which itself is at least several syndromes. Black people have 18 times more hypertensive kidney failure than white people which Tobian believes is due to a much lower potassium intake. Potassium protects against lesions of the kidney tubules, arteries, and glomeruli [Tobian]. As many as 15% of cases are thought to result from atherosclerotic renovascular disease from plaque build up on the kidney arteries, which in turn, along with glomerular derangement, may often be from a copper deficiency combined with a high salt intake [Moore]. Osteoarthritis itself probably does not cause kidney damage, but too much acetaminophen (Tylenol, Anacin-3, Liquiprin, Panadol. and Tempra) taken for it probably will. Tylenol also damages the liver. Since pain-killing drugs usually do not cure a disease, it is usually better to tolerate the pain if at all possible. An additional reason is that painkillers have been implicated as a risk factor in acquiring chronic fatigue syndrome (CFS, ME or CFIDS). I do not know which ones are implicated yet. One exception to adverse affects of pain medicines may be Methylsulfonylmethane (MSM). It is said to be fairly affective and virtually free of side effects. Pain, itself, can cause increased losses of potassium but I do not know if it can cause increased retention. I suspect not. People at risk, such as diabetics, should have regular urine and blood tests so that if small changes show up from the baseline they can be alerted to a much more serious underlying problem since kidney capacity is normally much more than we need and obvious problems are late in showing up. Systemic lupus erythmatosis (SLE or lupus) has caused such extensive damage to kidney tubules that the patients had chronic high plasma potassium which was not responsive to aldosterone [De Pronzo]. Since Lupus patients have been shown to have visibly damaged tubule in 66% of patients examined, the investigators believe that this hyperkalemia is more common than realized. Since Lupus is listed as one of the arthritic diseases and has some similar symptoms, there may be a temptation to use potassium supplements to heal it. Not only should this probably not be attempted, but also even foods high in potassium may be undesirable in the light of this report. Maybe with some lupus victims potassium intake may have a narrow safe range. Research to cast light on this would be highly desirable. Several circumstances have been found to act oppositely in rheumatoid arthritis from lupus such as pregnancy, estrogen, and schizophrenia [Mawson].

Other causes of high blood potassium are crush injury, severe burns, hemolysis (red blood cell destruction), hyperkalemic periodic paralysis (during paralysis episodes), acute tumor destruction after chemotherapy, transfusion of hemolyzed (aged) blood, Addison's disease (rare), hypoaldosteronism (very rare), severe dehydration, and respiratory acidosis. The last is a failure of the lungs to remove carbon dioxide leaving behind carbonic acid. Since acid (hydrogen and ammonium ion) interferes with potassium excretion, potassium can build up. Respiratory acidosis can result from failure of the lung to remove carbon dioxide because of bronchitis, asthma or airway obstruction. In this case, the high blood potassium can be mild or severe. People who have weak kidneys probably should sleep at night with the window open. In my opinion excessive dreaming is an indication of high carbon dioxide in the air. It is also conceivable that there is rarely such a thing as a 16alpha-18dihydroxy-deoxycorticosterone tumor analogous to aldosterone tumors. It would presumably cause potassium to be retained (see chapter 9). If such a tumor exists, I have not heard of it being reported.

There are several poisons and medications that can cause high blood potassium (hyperkalemia) for a short time after actual use. Angiotensin-converting enzyme (ACE) inhibitors {Captopril, Enalapril, Fosinopril}, non-steroid anti-inflammatory drugs (NSAIDs) {Indomethacin, Ibuprofen,

Ketorolac}, and potassium sparing diuretics {spironolactone, triamterene, amiloride} prevent excretion. The combined use of nonsteroidal anti-inflammatory drugs (NSAIDs) and beta-adrenergic blockers may increase the risk of life-threatening hyperkalemia [Kaufman p83] through their suppressive affect on the renin-aldosterone system, whereas the simultaneous administration of Lobenzaret (CCA) with NSAIDs through impairment of the renal tubular function [Ichinohe].

Medications which can cause too high a blood potassium are cyclosporine and lithium, by inhibiting prostaglandin stimulation of renin [Kaufman]. Cox-2 medicines for rheumatoid arthritis are said to have a damaging affect on kidney function. I do not know what the affect on potassium excretion is. Angiotensin receptor blockers such as Losartan, Valsartan, and Irbesartan, as well as the Candesartan and antiinfective agents Trimethoprim-sulfamethoxazole and pentamidine are said to be involved by a mechanism unknown to me. Digitalis glycosides, digoxin, and oleander (nerium oleander fluoride) inhibits the sodium/potassium cell wall pumps. Arginine (nuts and chocolate are very high in arginine), hypertonic solutions and salts cause cell leakage.

Fluoride damages the kidneys. The National Kidney Foundation has issued a warning against use of fluoridated water for dialysis. I do not know whether such damage causes potassium retention. However, fluoridated water should not be used for any purpose including bathing because fluoride causes brittle bones, damaged thyroid, dementia, and other damage. Aluminum accentuates some of the damage types such as dementia and kidney damage, so it is important not to use vaccines with aluminum in them [Gherardi], baking powder with aluminum in it, or aluminum pots and pans. You may see an extensive discussion on the awful side effects of fluoride in [http://tompetrie.net/id6.html]. We should make a concerted effort to get fluoride out of our water. The anticoagulant Heparin, alpha-adrenoreceptor stimulants, succinylcholine, and beta-adrenergic nerve blocking agents also produce high blood potassium. Acetaminophen damages the liver by degrading the detoxifier, glutathione peptide [http://www.xmission.com/~total/temple/Soapbox/Articles/glutathione.html] so it is possible that that is the mechanism for the kidneys also. If so, anyone who must take that drug should possibly increase cysteine (perhaps by means of whey), glutamate, and glycine in the diet, since those amino acids make up glutathione, and take as little as possible of the drug.

The kidneys are said to be a critical target organ for cadmium and this is especially ominous because the half-life of cadmium in the body is 17 years [World Health Organization p64]. I do not know if the damage affects potassium. In my opinion cadmium should not be used for plating screws or cathodic protection, and carpenters should not hold plated screws in the mouth.

Poisoning rarely causes severe high blood potassium directly unless the kidneys have been damaged or muscles destroyed as well. This is probably because of the high capacity of healthy kidneys.

There has also been proposed a rare, unknown genetic malfunction as a cause of hyperkalemia.

I believe that damage to the kidneys is the most common chronic problem. Ironically the kidneys can be damaged by a potassium deficiency with lesions of the distal portions of kidney and collecting ducts, which cause depression of renal concentrating ability [Epstein, p272] especially if high blood pressure is also involved [Tobian]. A deficiency state is very common in our society. Rubini believes that even a modest deficiency can cause irreversible kidney lesions [Rubini] in the collecting tubules, which is where the potassium is excreted. Some people with end stage kidney disease can have a total body cell deficit even though plasma potassium is normal [Knochel p450]. This is because when the cell potassium is low the body attempts to make the plasma potassium low also, in order that nerve impulses can continue to fire. So even though the plasma potassium seems normal, it is higher than the body would like it to be for nerve transmission in that case. Excess calcium can also damage the distal tubules of the kidneys with results the same as potassium deficiency [Epstein, p272]. It is possible that this is caused by an interference with magnesium absorption, which deficiency in turn prevents the potassium pumps from operating. It is said that excessive magnesium can damage the kidneys, especially for those who have poor kidney function to begin with. I do not know if any of those damages can directly cause damage of such a nature that potassium can not be excreted properly. However I would be greatly surprised if it did not at least contribute to making poison or other damage somewhat more severe since the effects of a potassium deficiency are very generalized and any decrease in the actual or working size of the kidneys should make other situations more difficult as well. Besides, in chronic kidney failure aldosterone secretion is often high and more potassium is excreted per unit of decreased glomerular filtration [Knochel p446]. This is probably because of increase of potassium pumps on the cell wall [Schon]. This is no doubt a considerable part of the reason why a large loss of kidney function must take place before adverse symptoms show up.

Persistent high blood pressure can damage the glomerulus, which is where the fluids from the blood are initially filtered into the kidney tubules. The most common glomerulus degeneration in the world is called Immunoglobulin A (IgA) nephropathy (IgAN) [Donadio]. Its progress can be muted by increasing ingestion of omega 3 oil in food [Donadio]. Walnuts are a source of omega

3 oil. The ratio of omega 6 to omega 3 should be one, but it is usually much higher in our society [Simopoulos]. I am not certain of what that kind of damage does to the potassium equilibrium. Probably it is not an important part of it by itself. Albumins in the urine are an indication of such damage. Early problems can only be detected by routine special tests on microalbinuria. People with insulin dependent diabetes should have such tests.

Immune stimulation by cytokine treatment (mainly interferon-alpha) involves several kinds of autoimmune renal diseases like acute interstitial nephritis or glomerulonephritis as well as interstitial and vascular rejection of renal transplants [Schwarz].

Aristolochic acid found in certain plants and botanicals (Stephania tetranddra, a Chinese slimming herb) is toxic to the kidneys and is a potential carcinogen. This chemical can cause serious kidney damage and the use of products that contain aristolochic acid has been associated with several occurrences of kidney failure. The American Food and Drug Administration has a program called MEDWATCH for people to report adverse reactions to untested substances, such as herbal remedies and vitamins; call 800-332-1088.

Never permit a radiological (x-ray) dye into your blood stream out of mere curiosity, but only if it is desperately important. A high percentage of people have kidney damage from such drugs, especially people with mild to moderate kidney impairment [Black] and over half of diabetics [Thompson]. In my opinion it is highly probable that healthy people have some hidden damage also, even in the absence of symptoms, from all the above substances. It is therefore not a good idea to use these drugs for trivial problems like pain, discomfort, reduction of a low fever (which should not be done anyway because fever is one of the body's defenses against infection), or for problems which can be solved in time with nutritious, non poisoned foods and healthy living or emotional support.

I do not know if diuretics can damage the kidneys. However there is a study which indicates that patients with kidney failure who are on diuretics had a higher death rate but also a higher rate of subsequent chronic kidney failure requiring dialysis. This may have been due to a potassium deficiency produced by the diuretics. The death rate was especially high in patients who failed to quickly respond to the diuretics with an increased flow of urine.

Other toxic agents that can damage kidneys include heavy metals like lead, arsenic (arsenic is given to chickens for worm control and gives young poultry meat 0.39 parts per million [Laskey]), and mercury (side effects of tooth amalgams), carbon tetrachloride (used in the dry cleaning industry), pesticides, and fungicides. Hydrocarbons are said to cause damage to the kidneys [Ravnskov]. I do not know which of these last poisons causes damage which prevents excretion and which prevents retention.

Lead probably prevents retention [in my opinion] and is the main cause of gout [Bateman] (see chapter 5). You would think that people suffering from gout would seldom have high blood potassium if I am correct, but I know of no evidence for such a correlation.

If there is a partial blockage of the urinary tract it can interfere with excreting potassium. Blockage would be most common in men because of the problem of swelling of the prostate tissue being common. I suspect that this prostate swelling is most often caused by a deficiency of the vitamins linoleic or linolenic acids (omega 6 and omega 3 oils) produced by the foolish custom of hydrogenating vegetable oils. I also suspect that it is sometimes caused by a zinc deficiency which in turn can be created by excessive intake of copper. Anyone having trouble with high potassium should have a urologist rule out prostate blockage as a source or contributor to the problem early on. It is also possible to check the matter oneself by inserting a catheter after urinating. If a significant amount of urine continues to come out there is an obstruction in the prostate or bladder opening. You have to be very careful and use good sterilization of both the catheter and as much of the organ as possible or bacteria can be introduced into the bladder and may be anyway. Bladder infections are difficult to get rid of although they are not usually dangerous. If there is an obstruction from swollen prostate it can usually be corrected surgically without the necessity of an abdominal incision. There are also hormone therapies which are said to be fairly effective for lesser prostate swellings.

Blockage is presumably possible from kidney stones. I do not know what affect this has on potassium. I do have some information on some of the causes. If calcium intake is normal but phosphorus is too low, calcium citrate stones can form [Sager]. On the other hand if phosphorus is much too high, say from drinking soft drinks, especially colas [Hall], calcium phosphate stones should form [I have no reference for this and am not sure it happens from soft drinks]. Stones are said to have an incidence as follows; calcium oxalate (65% - 75%), uric acid (7%), calcium phosphate (5%), cystine (2%), and ammonium phosphate (2%) stones. Uric acid stones are less probable when potassium was adequate in the diet in healthy people [Stewart].

CORRECTIVE PROCEDURES

There are some procedures available in a hospital that can provide some short term relief from a dangerous surge in blood potassium. Intravenous calcium, intravenous glucose and insulin [Schwartz 1978] will work for an hour or so. The calcium is probably effective because calcium inside kidney cells stimulate potassium excretion across collecting tubule membranes [Hunter]. Intravenous aldosterone will help the kidneys get rid of excess potassium.

Both in a hospital and at home, sodium bicarbonate will help considerably short term [Schwartz 1978] if there is any kidney function left, especially if the hyperkalemia is caused by acidosis (low blood alkalinity or pH), but is said to be dangerous if used for prolonged periods. It has been found that early or late administration of N-acetylcysteine (NAC) attenuates the progression of chronic renal failure in rats [Massola].

Drinking salt (sodium chloride) water as a vehicle for the bicarbonate is helpful. Increased urine flow increases potassium loss, so part of the effect of the salt solution may be from this phenomenon [Giebisch]. While sodium is a good antidote for high serum potassium, kidneys which have been conditioned by a prior low sodium intake can excrete an additionally larger amount of potassium from the collecting ducts than kidneys which have had a prior large intake. Furthermore, a low sodium intake causes higher potassium losses than an excessive sodium intake [Peterson 1977]. So it seems to me that a very low sodium intake normally would be the best way to go to avoid hyperkalemia. However I am not certain of this and in any case it may actually be the chloride that is involved.

Drinking extra water should be helpful, and indeed essential if dehydrated. However, drinking huge amounts of water (say a gallon) if severely dehydrated without sodium chloride is very dangerous and can kill you from hyponatremia (low sodium). Such dehydrated states should be relieved slowly and combined with some sodium chloride salt, as well as some potassium chloride in the case of normal people with adequate kidney function. Oral rehydration therapy (ORT salts) is in order for people with adequate kidney function. Of course it is best not to become dehydrated in the first place. Too yellow a urine has been proposed as a symptom of dehydration. However this cue can not be used if you have been taking iboflavin (vitamin B-2) supplements, since that vitamin turns the urine a bright yellow. You may see an extensive discussion of water in [http://www.who.int/water_sanitation_health/dwq/nutrientsindw.pdf]

You may see a discussion of drugs to correct hyperkalemia (but aldosterone is not discussed) along with doses, contraindications, symptoms, tests, and ECG charts at this site [http://www.emedicine.com/emerg/topic261.htm]. Also flurocortisone acetate (FCA), has been found to increase potassium excretion without many other changes [Furuya]. If this is happening by release of potassium from the cells, it is a dangerous procedure. If drinking extra water is prescribed and you gag on pure water, adding extra water to your soup and using two thirds of fruit juice as water (although I do not recommend fruit juice routinely during kidney failure because of a high potassium content relative to its other nutrition) should help. You would immediately think that reducing the amount of potassium which you eat was in order long term and this is, indeed, usually prescribed. The main problem is that potassium tends to be correlated with other essential nutrients. However an immediate gain can be achieved by cutting out foods unusually high in potassium per calorie such as celery (see second table in chapter 14). It would seem to be in order to cut out foods moderate in potassium per calorie that are rather low in other nutrients such as apple juice. Increasing intake of foods unusually high in other nutrients such as wheat germ and liver (liver if uric acid is normal) would no doubt solve part of the above problem.

Chitosan has been found to have a profoundly advantageous affect on people with kidney failure by an unknown mechanism [Jing], but these researchers do not give information on potassium in their abstract.

It is entirely possible that it would be desirable to take vitamin and mineral supplements as well when afflicted high blood potassium. If so, be sure they are complete and balanced as a rule, excepting if you know you are low in one or two. Dangerous imbalances are possible otherwise. In particular, unless you get copper at about one-seventh the amount of zinc, you could suffer from a severe copper deficiency with hemorrhoids, slipped or herniated discs, and aneurysms (which cause strokes in the brain) some of the most dangerous symptoms. The reverse is also true for copper's affect on zinc with adverse symptoms, such as swollen prostate, although they are somewhat less immediately dangerous symptoms. You should keep in mind that no vitamin capsules have adequate amounts of the macro nutrients such as potassium, calcium, magnesium, sodium, chloride, phosphate, and amino acids, so imbalances are possible even if the tablet is balanced with what micro nutrients it does contain.

Wine can be obtained without sulfites but because it has a poison in it which interferes with potassium excretion [McDonald], wine should not be used during high blood potassium. I have no information as to whether this poison has been identified and ethanol itself is said to increase excretion [McDonald]. However by all means cut out wine and alcoholic beverages fermented with sulfur dioxide whether potassium is high or not and cut them out with or without sulfur dioxide during high blood potassium. I do not know how potent the affect is, but there is no point testing the matter on yourself. Wine has been proposed as good for the heart in normal people, but if the mechanism for this goodness is retardation of potassium excretion, I suggest that getting adequate potassium is a superior strategy for kidney intact people and not getting overwhelming amounts of vitamin B-1 from pills. There is no good substitute for nutritious, unprocessed food free of poison, for then you do not usually have to scratch your head over how to balance things. When the protein in meat, eggs, and milk is burned for energy the nitrogen in it degrades to ammonium, uric acid, and urea. Damaged kidneys can have trouble excreting these wastes also. The trouble is direct for potassium excretion since ammonium is excreted by the same cells that excrete potassium, so potassium excretion is interfered with. For this reason people with damaged kidneys are often urged not to eat excessive amounts of high protein foods. A trial suggests that 0.6 gram of protein per kilogram of body weight slows down progression of kidney disease [D'Amico]. This would be roughly less than 50 grams for a lean 150-pound person. There may be an additional reason so far as potassium is concerned. When the body suffers from a potassium deficiency the kidneys activate an enzyme which degrades glutamic acid. This seems to me to be an adaptation to conserve potassium by interfering with excretion at the excretion site. It may be that extra ammonium in the body may interfere somewhat as well, not something desirable when suffering from an excess of potassium. It is probable also that the ammonium can act as if it were potassium so far as nerve conduction is concerned because it has the same size and charge which would make the situation even worse than the potassium value itself would seem to indicate. I know of no experimental evidence which would cast light on ammonium in the blood in nerve conduction though. In any case it is fairly important in the long run not to remove meat, milk and eggs from the diet completely since these foods provide amino acids lysine and methionine, which plants are low in. I suspect that the equivalent of the weight of an egg at each meal would be adequate for mature normal people. They also provide vitamin B-12 although that is easy to provide with pills. Pills should be safe except when relieving a vitamin B-12 deficiency. When doing this a potassium supplement would be in order because the surge in red blood cell metabolism can withdraw potassium so rapidly from the blood plasma that it can be life threatening [Lawson]. An additional argument is often advanced against using meat, liver, and eggs because of the anti cholesterol fad. It is very unlikely that dietary cholesterol is an important part of the problem, but rather excessive synthesis within the body. Cholesterol has only gone up in the diet from 683 to 734 milligrams between 1909 and 1961 and the Masai tribe has low cholesterol [Brown p8] in spite of a high meat diet. If the problem is most often caused by low copper [Carr] as I suspect, warning against eating shellfish or liver is exaggerating the problem, not helping, because those foods are high in copper. So be sure to get a small amount of high quality protein at every meal, or at least within 2 hours of a meal. If your cholesterol is high, make sure the protein is not milk, which is low in copper or supplement copper. But supplement copper moderately, perhaps 2 milligrams per day, especially moderately if you have diabetes (see chapter 6).

Glucosamine is currently being touted as advantageous for some of the arthritis diseases. I have a suspicion that part of its efficacy may be due to it furnishing glutamine for ammonium synthesis in the kidneys for ammonia production goes up and potassium excretion goes down when ingesting glutamine [Tannen p458]. If so, I suspect that taking this material should be counter productive and therefore contraindicated during high blood potassium, and perhaps food containing large amounts of it also. I do not have information about glutamine in food.

Acids which can be absorbed but not burned (metabolized) will interfere with potassium excretion since hydrogen ion competes with potassium at the excretion site. Unfortunately I do not know which foods are involved. However, I do suspect vinegar (acetic acid) since vinegar has been suggested as being advantageous for rheumatoid arthritis, which I am convinced is accentuated by a potassium deficiency. Acetic acid can be metabolized [Winegrad] but it could be that much of it is excreted before entering the cells or that well-fed people do not burn it all. Cherries and cranberries fall into this same suspicion also (however researchers have proposed antioxidants responsible for the affect of cherries on rheumatoid arthritis and gout), cranberries because I have heard they increase urine acidity (but no hard evidence). I am almost certain that the citric acid in citrus fruit is burnt in the body since citric acid is part of the Kreb's cycle so I assume that citrus fruits are safe. It is possible that the low metabolism during the night could prevent citrate from being burnt, and thus make susceptible people more prone to headaches and potassium retention. It would be a good idea for researchers to perform experiments to determine this for sure or to make the information well known if it has already been done since a little fruit like citrus should be reasonable if a patient's potassium overage is mild and the low nutrition value of fruit would not be a major problem in that case.

Of course potassium supplements, salt substitutes, ORT salts, some athletic drinks, and potassium-based baking powders must not be used at all if you have high blood potassium, except possibly during virulent diarrhea.

Because aldosterone suffers a drastic decline during dehydration it is important that you drink more water than just barely enough to satisfy thirst. Aldosterone is the hormone the body relies on to excrete potassium when the sodium intake is low. Furthermore extra water probably makes it easier for the kidneys to unload potassium. Perspiration should help considerably to remove excess potassium also, but only if it is not allowed to dehydrate the body, for perspiration contains potassium. I am not certain beyond a doubt that this is a wise way to augment kidney function, but it sounds at least reasonably safe. Sweat glands are not nearly as efficient at retaining vital materials as kidneys. Saunas should enable perspiration. You may see some theory about saunas here and a link to how to construct various kinds of saunas in that same site [http://www.drlwilson.com/articles/sauna_therapy.htm]. . Enemas also cause large potassium losses [Dunning]. Leaving water in contact with the mucous membranes for a long time increases the losses. I do not know whether this is a desirable strategy routinely or not, but I should think it would be helpful in an emergency at least.

Licorice has a chemical, glycyrrhetinic acid, in it which interferes with degradation of aldosterone, so licorice (but not the licorice candy, which is said to be anise seed extract) should be a reasonably safe temporary palliative. I do not know if long term use is desirable or not. The fact that licorice also increases cortisol indicates that it probably is not. The same degradation is said to be true of grapefruit. I do not know what the status of other citrus fruits is. Aldosterone injection is excellent for increasing survival in metabolic shock, but amounts must be kept between 0.2 and 0.4 milligrams per kilogram of body weight in rats [Schumer]. This last would only be available in a hospital of course. It may be that deoxycorticosterone (DOC) would be better for people eating too much salt (see chapter 9).

Because acid interferes with potassium excretion, it should not be surprising that bicarbonate of soda (baking powder) causes large potassium loss. This also should be a reasonably safe temporary palliative. Whether it is safe as a routine strategy or not, I do not know. Sodium bicarbonate is often used as baking powder, but this is not necessarily a good idea routinely. It has recently been questioned as to being of any help in life threatening high blood potassium, but I find this hard to believe except maybe in almost complete loss of kidney function. Caffeine has been proposed as tending toward low blood potassium I do not know whether it is a good idea or not.

Hyperventilating (breathing rapidly) gets rid of carbon dioxide (carbonic acid) via the lungs to an abnormal extent. This should be an advantageous procedure to know if you are in a taxicab on the way to a hospital to treat metabolic potassium shock. I have no knowledge of it being tried, but I would have thought it should help temporarily to avoid a lethal ending.

I do not know for sure what value potassium must attain before drastic remedial action should be taken. I suspect that over 6.0 meq per liter is necessary to start to threaten actual death. However attempting to alleviate the problem nutritionally until the underlying problem is discovered should be inherently fairly safe and without a doubt almost always a desirable additional strategy at least. See table 2 in chapter 14 for potassium in food in descending concentration order.

It is good sense to forego processed food, alcohol, and tobacco in order to stay as healthy as possible even when that garbage is not the direct cause of the disease you are trying to avoid. What little phony pleasure, financial advantage, or excitement that garbage gives you is much more than counter balanced by the pain and misery that garbage ultimately brings, in my opinion. It would be better to attempt to attain happiness with camaraderie or good jokes.

CHAPTER 8
POTASSIUM SUPLEMENTATION

SUMMARY

This chapter discusses the interactions of potassium supplements with magnesium and vitamin B-1. It explores the utility of the various forms of potassium supplementation such as sodium free table salt, glucosamine, vegetable juices, tablets and solutions, sodium free baking powder, water softeners, and fertilizer. Some inadequate supplements are also discussed such as sea salt and athletic drinks.

Potassium is the most dangerous of the essential nutrients. While mild chronic overdoses are probably not damaging, because of the efficiency of the kidneys in clearing excesses, a very large acute overdose can be extremely dangerous if not cleared in time. As little as 8 to 10 thousand milligrams of potassium taken suddenly can give nausea. A teaspoonful of potassium salt contains about 3300 milligrams of potassium. As little as 14,000 milligrams of potassium taken suddenly can cause death in some replete people, especially those who normally have a low intake for long periods prior. Therefore, one may not use supplements without regard to any caution. However the main reason I do not recommend supplements is because normally it is quite possible to receive all the potassium you need from food, and this source is inherently safe [Sebastian], inexpensive, and with reasonable wisdom, balanced with respect to other nutrients. Food as a source usually results in shorter hospital stays than supplements [Norris]. My recommendation against supplements is based primarily on concern of an imbalance with other nutrients rather than any likely chance of an acute overdose. The Institute of Medicine does not set an upper limit from food because there is no evidence of chronic excess potassium in healthy individuals.

The imbalance that I know of which is probably most dangerous is the imbalance with thiamine (vitamin B-1) if animal experiments are an indication. If potassium supplements are given during the wet heart disease of beriberi (thiamine deficiency) it is very dangerous. See chapter 3 for an extensive discussion. Also see chapter 6 if you have diabetes. If potassium supplements are given, it is very important that the vitamin B-1 intake must be adequate at the same time.

All purpose vitamin capsules contain no potassium but usually contain vitamin B-1. Some contain 1000% of the recommended daily intake and one even contains 5000%. This is probably dangerous for most heart disease in the absence of adequate potassium in food or supplements.

The recent discovery that something in vegetables, especially onions, prevents bones from losing density [Muhlbauer & Li] is just one more hint that we can not use supplements instead of food with complete assurance that there is no other advantage from good food.

I am also concerned about liability were I to recommend supplements and someone were to have real or imagined difficulties. However there are a few times when supplements would be desirable, sometimes even imperative and life saving. Severe diarrhea is one such a time. Cholera is an especially lethal diarrhea and oral rehydration therapy (ORT salts) is in order. ORT salts are a mixture of salts containing sodium, chloride, potassium, and bicarbonate. The Lancet journal has stated that ORT therapy is the most important medical advance of the 20th century. Diarrhea causes more deaths to children than any other infectious disease [http://www.rehydrate.org/rehydration/index. html]. It has been suggested that supplementation with potassium would be in order for cirrhosis of the liver also [Conn]. Potassium bicarbonate has been used to correct the acidic serum associated with diabetes [Soler]. It has been found to increase the density of bone [Sebastian] by virtue of decreased calcium losses in urine [http://jn.nutrition.org/content/123/9/1623.full.pdf]. Potassium citrate also increases the density of bone [Jehle], almost certainly by the same mechanisms. Severe emotional stress and emotional stress of surgery might be two other occasions when supplementation would be in order. Also, a low potassium to sodium ratio has been shown to be a risk factor for cancer [Jansson], and increases the incidence of calcium kidney stones [Stamler], and bronchitis [Schwartz]. Potassium supplements decreases the risk of stroke [Green]. All these are in the presence of inadequate diets, no doubt.

Rarely acute hypokalemic paralysis afflicts people and can be life threatening. The symptoms are weakness, low plasma potassium, progressing to paralysis. Most cases are due to familial hypokalemic paralysis; however, a few cases are associated with diverse underlying causes including thyrotoxic periodic paralysis from hyper active thyroid, barium poisoning, renal tubular acidosis, primary hyperaldosteronism, licorice ingestion, and gastrointestinal potassium losses. Immediate potassium replacement is in order coupled with an aggressive search for the underlying cause [http://www.ithyroid.com/ potassium.htm] [Stedwell]. If urine potassium is low in the above syndrome, correction must be with small amounts of potassium chloride to avoid rebound hyperkalemia because this is an indication that urine is low because of inappropriate movement of potassium into cells [Lin].

More than 20 % of the people who are hospitalized have plasma potassium content lower than 3.6 milliequivalents per liter (which they define as hypokalemia) [Gennari]. It would no doubt be considerably higher a percentage if an accurate figure could be obtained for people with rheumatoid arthritis, who lose potassium from their platelets when blood is withdrawn, and if there never was a delay in analyzing the blood. So such people would probably be better off with reasonable supplementation since hospital food is usually low in potassium and that low a potassium content in plasma is dangerous even if correct and near the upper figure. Potassium replacement recommended in medical texts (a maximum rate of infusion of 0.3-0.5 milliequivalents per killigrams of body weight per hour and a maximum daily replacement of 3-5 milliequivalents per kilogram of body weight may be inadequate for profound hypokalaemia (less than 11.5 millequivalents per liter of plasma) Maybe it should be 3-4 times as great [Welfare].

A review of potassium by Feng and MacGregor has concluded that increased potassium will lower blood pressure, prevent renal damage, reduce calcium excretion and kidney stones, reduce the risk of type 2 diabetes, cardiac arrhythmias, and stroke independently of blood pressure affects [https://www.ncbi.nlm.nih.gov/pmc/articles/PMC1121081/].

MAGNESIUM

The status of magnesium is especially important because potassium can not be absorbed efficiently if magnesium is deficient [Petersen] [MacIntyre] [Manitius] [Dawson]. One person reports getting red cell magnesium up to normal with magnesium orotate and Epsom sulfate foot baths every other day, along with choline citrate supplement in the hope the last helps with absorption. Magnesium as the sulfate is a poor source and can even be dangerous. Magnesium as the orotate has been shown to be more readily absorbed than the carbonate [Schlebusch]. Athletes had there swimming, cycling and running times decreased in the magnesium-orotate group compared with the controls and their insulin system markedly affected [Golf]. The orotate is probably having an affect physiologically in its own right, and is most likely not making the magnesium more soluble or acting as a chelating agent. 400

milligrams of magnesium per day is the amounts usually recommended. See Rude's article for safe use of magnesium clinically [Rude].

Processing removes 75% of the magnesium, which, combined with sugar, phosphates, alcohol, stress and high fat diets that increase magnesium deficiency, is said to cause a deficiency in 80% of the population [Rogers]. Magnesium is needed in order to power the ATPase [Hamil-Ruth] because potassium can not be absorbed effectively during a magnesium deficit [Kohvakka]. It takes six months for the sodium/potassium pumps to return toward normal after a magnesium deficiency is corrected [Anonymous], so the magnesium must be an integral part of the pumps.

A test for magnesium deficiency is to inject 2.4 milligrams of magnesium per kilogram of body weight over 4 hours and urine collected for 24 hours. If 25% of the magnesium is retained a deficiency is probable. If 50% of the magnesium is retained a deficiency is certain [Rude].

SODIUM FREE TABLE SALT

Sodium free table salt is the means usually used for supplementation of heart disease patients. The original justification for this was to provide for the psychic dependence on a salty taste without providing sodium. So medical men thought, since people will satisfy their craving for salty flavor whether we warn them against it or not, we will give them the salty flavor without the sodium. Since the chloride provides the salty taste this was easy. Just substitute another positively charged atom for sodium. This philosophy carried to its logical conclusion led them even to use lithium as a substitute atom. It was then that lithium's pronounced properties as a tranquilizer became evident.

Potassium was considered inert, or largely so. In addition to potassium, ammonium and choline molecules were also used. These molecules may not be useless. Choline is a biologically active material similar to vitamins but made by the body. Some men may require more than others because six out of twenty six suffered muscle damage and increased liver lipid content when receiving inadequate choline [Penry p192]. Betaine is derived from choline in the body, which betaine furnishes a methyl group to convert homocysteine to methionein [Penry p 197]. It is thought to be adequate in unprocessed food. Coffee, beer, potatoes, and oranges have significant amounts. There is an article that gives concentrations of choline and betaine in common foods [Zeisel]. They say that choline is important for normal membrane function, acetylcholine synthesis and methyl group metabolism; the choline requirement for humans is 550 mg/d for men (adequate intake). Betaine, a choline derivative, is important because of its role in the donation of methyl groups to homocysteine to form methionine. In tissues and foods, there are multiple choline compounds that contribute to total choline concentration (choline, glycerophosphocholine, phosphocholine, phosphatidylcholine and sphingomyelin). In their study, they collected representative food samples and analyzed the choline concentration of 145 common foods using liquid chromatography-mass spectrometry. Foods with the highest total choline concentration (mg/100 g) were: beef liver (418), chicken liver (290), eggs (251), wheat germ (152), bacon (125), dried soybeans (116) and pork (103). The foods with the highest betaine concentration (mg/100 g) were: wheat bran (1339), wheat germ (1241), spinach (645), pretzels (237), shrimp (218) and wheat bread (201). A number of epidemiologic studies have examined the relationship between dietary folic acid and cancer or heart disease.. Choline is said to enhance the salt (chloride) taste. Short term it is said to enhance memory in young people and in babies from choline adequate mothers. Choline supplements increase memory ability in baby rats when administered either before or after being born, probably from an increase in brain cell size [Williams 1998]. Its long-term effects as a supplement are unknown to me.

Ammonium, at least, may interfere with potassium excretion if it is absorbed in the intestines and has been used to protect the kidneys [Selye 1945]. So far as I know the substitutes above are reasonably harmless for healthy people who have normal blood pressure. Ammonium is even synthesized by the kidneys during a potassium deficiency from glutamine, and this is probably a strategy of the body, the purpose of which is to prevent potassium loss. Eating glutamine increases ammonia excretion and decreases potassium excretion [Tannen, p458]. However, if ammonium chloride is used during a potassium deficiency a dangerous taurine depletion occurs resulting in lethal heart disease in cats [Dow] so it would be a good idea to avoid it for humans until more is known.

Potassium enriched table salt almost halved the mortality from cardiovascular disease of retired men studied in China over a 31 month period [Chang], so potassium deficiency must be a cause of or is considerably accentuating some other cause in half the heart disease in China. I suspect the fraction would be found to be higher yet in the USA if whole body potassium were ever determined routinely here.

Sulfate is an excretory product, so the sulfate as the anion with potassium should be, at the least, useless, but I know of no evidence. Adding potassium sulfate to a processed food diet should have the same effect as adding sulfuric acid to a normal diet, whatever that is. In any case, sulfate and phosphate increases potassium excretion [Giebisch]. Phosphate causes 100% mortality in people suffering from heart disease.

GLUCOSAMINE

That synthesis of ammonium just mentioned may be part of the reason that glucosamine has shown evidence of being useful for arthritics, especially osteoarthritis [http://www.arthritis-glucosamine.net/article-etail.php?ID=33]. Glucosamine is a biological reaction product of glutamine and glucose. The rationale usually given is that this provides a molecule which is incorporated into connecting tissue. Glucosamine is a combination of fructose-6-phosphate sugar and glutamic acid and is provided in supplements as the sulfate. Glucosaminec breaks down forming ammonium ion in the body, so it is possible that it is getting part of its beneficial results by virtue of providing ammonium ion in the kidneys as well as hydrogen ion from the sulfate, which interferes with potassium excretion (but keep in mind that I have no evidence yet that osteoarthritis is caused or accentuated by a potassium deficiency, and probably is not directly involved). If so, glucosamine could be considered a potassium supplement of sorts, also. Glutamine or glutamic acid is a major transporter of nitrogen, transporting one third of nitrogen [Labow p1503] and is presumably useful in that role. Therefore it seems to me that this would be a poor substitute for adequate potassium. Labow claims that the less than 10 grams per day usually eaten should be increased to 20 to 40 grams for those under stress, and that it considerably increases survival of hospital patients and should in addition be part of intravenous feeding [Labow p 1503,1510]. Conserving potassium may be part of its efficacy. It is apparently used to help excrete acid since glutaminase and glutamine consumption are both increased by acidosis [Labow p1504]. Glutaminedipeptide is more soluble and has a longer shelf life than glutamine [Labow p1509]. Some commercial glucosamine products are also a potassium supplement, since they contain large amounts of potassium chloride.

You can tell which materials are present in a product by the list of ingredients. The materials of highest concentration are supposed to be placed at the beginning of the list. Select the substitute, which has potassium nearest the beginning of the list in order to avoid the small chance of side effects of the other ingredients should you decide to use supplements unless you are sure you need the other ingredients also. Ingredients of some clinical supplements are given in a book by Friedberg [Friedberg p348].

VEGETABLE LIQUERS

Green coconut milk has been proposed as a potassium supplement for cholera patients [Carpenter]. I assume that celery or bamboo shoot juice would have a similar value. If used for diarrhea it is important that salt and perhaps bicarbonate of soda be eaten at the same time in amounts approximating

ORT salts. Such a juice strategy would probably be not quite as effective or at least able to be controlled as potassium chloride or ORT salts, but might be all that is available at times for some people. Vegetable juice is much higher in potassium per Calorie than the original vegetable. So it has some of the characteristics of a supplement.

TABLETS AND LIQUIDS

There is a liquid supplement in which the bitter taste of potassium is masked by cherry extract. It is conceivable that a child could get a fatal overdose in this form. Non of the other above concoctions are substantially more dangerous than other household items like aspirin, for instance. I would recommend against storing potassium in an easy to eat form in general, however. Liquids containing more than 390 milligrams of potassium must have a prescription in order to be sold in the USA. 100 milligrams is the limit for tablets.

Enteric tablets are also available. These are tablets that will not dissolve until they reach the intestines. Since there are no pain nerves in the intestines as in the stomach, you are not distracted by the commotion that ensues when they suddenly create a saturated potassium chloride solution near the intestine wall, as you would be if they dissolved in the stomach, which has pain nerves. Gastric release tablets give a bad stomachache on an empty stomach. There have been cases [Baker] reported of enteric tablets becoming caught in the fold of the intestines and causing ulcers, some even fatal, when the enteric coating dissolved. You can eat these tablets with safety so far as ulcers are concerned by chewing them while drinking a glass of juice. The bitter taste is largely eliminated also. Of course tablets are an expensive way to increase potassium.

A new enteric tablet has been developed which is prescribed by 99% or more of the doctors today. It is called "slo-release". It is designed to release its potassium slowly so that no portion of the digestive tract is overwhelmed with a concentrated solution. It is probably as reasonably safe as anything is in this dangerous world [Palva] [Block]. The safest of all would be to also chew these tablets with juice. The American law prevents more than 100 milligrams of potassium in each one, so that seven or more must be taken with each meal to double the potassium intake of a junk food diet in order to bring it up to a very healthy diet. At least two at each meal would be necessary to bring junk food to a passable intake.

There is also a liquid that contains tiny enteric particles containing potassium chloride. This is only available by prescription. It should be similar to Slo release enteric tablets and should be inherently safe against ulceration, but not against overdose.

Potassium gluconate comes in a tablet that can be chewed with juice also. Since gluconate is metabolized in the body, this form should be similar in its effects to potassium from plants or from the bicarbonate (bicarbonate to be discussed later with sodium free baking powder). Women afflicted by premenstrual syndrome were cured within 4 cycles by 800 milligrams per day of potassium as the gluconate [Takacs]. Potassium has been prescribed as the aspartate usually with magnesium for heart disease. I do not know what the rationale for using the aspartate anion is, although the ammonium excretion system may be involved. Also potassium moves into the cell more easily as the aspartate [Ring]. However both magnesium and potassium are absorbed more effectively as the chloride than as the aspartate [Classen]. Healthy people are probably best advised to get amino acids for endurance from food [Williams]. Indeed as much as possible of all essential nutrients should be gotten from unprocessed food.

JUICE

There is a safety advantage in keeping your taste in touch with potassium supplement. Potassium chloride dissolved in fruit juice gives it a fine, rich flavor in reasonable amounts. Potassium bicarbonate gives it a delightful tang. When too much is put in, the flavor becomes nauseating and bitter. Thus you have a built in safeguard. Another inherent safeguard is the presence of adequate water. Potassium supplementation is especially dangerous during dehydration, as will be mentioned in chapter 9 and 12, because of a drastic decline of aldosterone during dehydration. The use of juice reduces danger during dehydration somewhat. Even so, supplements should not be taken until at least an hour after dehydration has been largely corrected using some sodium salt supplement to avoid dangerous low blood sodium, in order to give aldosterone a chance to be secreted again. An additional advantage of juice in conjunction with potassium is that it can be more readily taken between meals. Potassium can be more readily absorbed then because it does not tend to form an overload combined with potassium in food. That also probably makes it less dangerous for people with weak hearts or kidneys. People with very weak kidneys leading to high blood potassium should be under a doctor's care and should not take potassium supplements on their own, or at all (see chapter 7). In addition, between meals probably provides minimum interference with other nutrient absorption, such as that of magnesium. For a similar reason it is probably advantageous to divide meals into more than three per day when recovering from a deficiency [Fabry].

SODIUM FREE BAKING POWDER

Sodium free baking powder is a supplement also, including those times when used for baking. It is potassium as the bicarbonate or tartrate. Dissolved in fruit juice, the bicarbonate gives it a delightful tang like soda pop soft drinks as mentioned in "JUICE". The bicarbonate has been shown to be not as effective as the ehloride in relieving a deficiency both as to reducing cell sodium content and raising plasma levels of potassium [Giebisch] [DeLand].. It is the chloride in sodium table salt that causes high blood pressure because sodium bicarbonate lowered blood pressure 5 mm of mercury while sodium chloride had no affect [Luft], possibly because sodium chloride was already high in their diet. Even so, potassium chloride reduces blood pressure in sodium loaded spontaneously hypertensive rats and protects them from kidney damage [Ellis]. Any designation of high blood pressure must be by comparing the pressure to the average among low sodium chloride intake people [Tekol]. Both sodium and chloride are necessary for pressure augmentation [Boegshold]. This phenomenon may be involved with 18hydroxy-deoxycorticosterone steroid hormone (18OH-DOC) because that hormone is raised in one of the at least three forms of high blood pressure and that hormone is the hormone used by the body to increase acid excretion (see chapter 9). However, kidney lesions are prevented by potassium chloride supplements by an unknown mechanism [Ellis], and such lesions are the most important effects of high blood pressure. Aneurysms are important also, but these are almost certainly will not appear if copper is adequate in the diet, for healthy, copper nourished blood vessels take ten times as much pressure as normal in order to rupture. While potassium chloride raises blood pressure somewhat, if potassium is low it would still be desirable to raise potassium if deficient with that supplement or some other supplement because 3% of white people with 4.1 milliequivalents of potassium in blood plasma have high blood pressure while this goes down progressively to 1% for 4.8 [Walsh]. Diets low in sodium chloride and high in potassium, magnesium and calcium are associated with freedom from high blood pressure [He]. Actually it is the chloride associated with the sodium that is the problem as mentioned above, not the sodium itself. Sodium alone has no affect, or causes blood pressure to fall. For a review of the affect of numerous nutrients on blood pressure, see Houston [Houston].

Potassium bicarbonate decreases losses of calcium in the urine significantly. It is twice as effective as potassium chloride in doing so [Frassetto 2000]. As a result, potassium bicarbonate prevents osteoporosis (bone loss) and calcium kidney stones [Morris]. The key trigger for bone loss is blood pH (alkalinity). There is no loss at pH = 7.4, but bone loss becomes increasingly severe below that until it plateaus at pH = 6.8 [Arnett]. The main key to keeping blood at pH = 7.4 is potassium in food unassociated with chloride or animal derived acid generating food [Arnett].

Potassium bicarbonate also has the attribute of preventing muscle mass degradation in post menopausal women [Frassetto 1997].

If any kind of baking powder is used, it is important that it not contain aluminum. Aluminum is a poison and is suspected to cause a disease similar to Alzheimer's disease [Masters]. It is synergistic with (reinforce each other) the poisonous fluoride [Varner] often foolishly put into municipal water. Aluminum also causes surface bone resorption in mammals and navicular disease in horses [http://george-eby-research.com/html/nav.html]. Fluoride in city water causes fluorosis discoloration of teeth, weakened bones, damage to the kidneys and immune system, low thyroid secretion, and, worst of all, damage to the nerves resembling Alzheimer's disease, So does fluoride in insecticide on food.

You may acquire pure potassium bicarbonate for as little as $10 or less per pound in three pound purchases by putting "potassium bicarbonate" into Google's shopping feature. That will give you well over a million milligrams, so will last a long time. Just be sure you store it out of reach of children.

The phosphate is probably similar to the bicarbonate in regard to being absorbed. Phosphate is probably very dangerous for those with heart disease. Excess phosphate has caused 100 per cent mortality during heart disease [Selye 1958]. Soft drinks often contain phosphoric acid.

I have taken potassium as the bicarbonate for several weeks when I was young without any obvious great difficulty. I did have the strong feeling during that time that I was more susceptible to muscle cramps. However this was probably a function of too little calcium or vitamin D at the same time or even more likely a low cell potassium since potassium as the bicarbonate should not be substantially different from potassium in food unless food anions temporarily prevent plasma alkalosis. Calcium supplements will probably solve the problem. If in the unlikely possibility that the bicarbonate should prove in the future to be not, on balance, be a desirable method of relieving a deficiency, then it follows that it may be desirable to go back to the use of yeast for leavening bread. The bicarbonate should be close to equivalent to potassium acquired from food, though. Sodium bicarbonate is very undesirable for leavening because it is basic. Potassium is extremely sensitive to hydrogen ion, and sodium bicarbonate can triple excretion, as discussed in chapter 9. Even hyperventilating (breathing too hard) will have an equivalent affect on excretion (this would probably make a good emergency procedure in the case of high potassium shock if a hospital can not be reached or on the way to the hospital as mentioned in chapter 7). The overall effects from potassium tartrate in baking powder would probably depend on whether the tartrate is metabolized or not and this I do not know.

The bicarbonate may be indicated in renal tubular acidosis [Morgan] and for gout (see chapter 5). It is also said to be desirable to have either part of the sodium as the bicarbonate in ORT salts during diarrhea and dehydration or an equivalent amount with the potassium.

WATER SOFTENING SALTS

When potassium salts are used to soften water, significant amounts of extra potassium will be added to one's intake if the water is hard and much of the water is used. It may be that water softener potassium salt would provide an inexpensive supplement. However it would be difficult to control the amount ingested. Such salts must be kept guarded from children because of severe scarring of the stomach, including obstruction of the outlet, and metabolic acidosis from eating the salts [Mosely]. I assume this is true for other potassium salts containing chloride also.

COMBINATION TABLE SALTS

For some time now the main table salt suppliers have placed on the market a table salt that contains both potassium and sodium. Two brands which I am familiar with are Morton's "LITE" salt and Sterling's "LO-SALT" or "HALF and HALF". There is also "HALF SALT" from Canadian Salt Co., a sister company to Morton Salt Co. There is a potassium chloride table salt on the market that contains lysine to mask the potassium flavor [http://www.alsosalt. com/nutritionfacts.html]. I do not know what the long term affects of lysine would be, but it should be marvelous when suffering from certain viruses such as chicken pox, shingles, genital herpes, roseola, and fever sores because lysine helps to mute the effects of the virus, significantly reducing the occurrence (when taken routinely during the disease), severity, and healing time of herpes simplex virus [Griffith]. You can recognize the herpes shingles virus by large patches of a painful rash that appears on one side of the body in people under emotional stress , older people, or people whose immune system has been compromised. If you must have the salty taste of the chloride these brands would be a fairly reasonable way to go. In the case of diarrhea they would, I suspect, be the best way other than the ORT salts mentioned above. In many areas of the undeveloped countries they may be the only way. They have not caught on much in the developed countries, I suppose because the diarrheas are not often fatal in the temperate regions, possibly because potassium is less often lost in perspiration, or because the tropical diarrheas are more virulent. That greater virulence of tropical diseases is no doubt the main reason why tropical countries are often referred to by the euphemistic term "developing". The potassium table salts containing sodium are more intrinsically safe from an overdose than pure potassium salts. On balance, though, the possible long term effect of the sodium chloride on hypertension would be sufficiently disadvantageous to make their routine use undesirable except in moderate amounts for sodium must be combined with chloride to raise blood pressure. Sodium alone, as the bicarbonate or probably as citrate also, lowers blood pressure [McCarty]. Also I have a suspicion based on personal experience that potassium chloride can accentuate pain from some other cause. but I have no proof. It may be eventually shown that the best way would be a salt that contains many essential minerals, including magnesium, calcium, potassium and trace elements and other anions, including bicarbonate and especially iodide, in addition to a reasonable amount of chloride. Currently I am aware of no supporting theory nor of anything in supermarkets or health food stores similar to this last, although Cardia contains magnesium and lysine. Research should be performed to shed light on this considering that most people put salt on their food. The above existing combination salts usually contain about one atom of potassium to two of sodium.

It is possible that combination table salts should also be kept out of the reach of children in view of the affect that water softener salts had on the child mentioned above.

SEA SALT

Sea salt is not a source of potassium. Even if the salt is obtained by evaporating seawater to dryness, it will still only contain about 4% of potassium salts. Sea salt is really only a sodium table salt no matter how it is made. In addition it has the potential of retaining all the mercury and other poisons contained in seawater if evaporated to dryness, which could be a disadvantage.

DEAD SEA SALT

The Dead Sea water has a reputation for healing rheumatoid arthritis and has been successfully investigated with healing lasting up to three months [Sukenik]. It has two and a half to ten times as much potassium chloride by weight as sodium chloride and an even greater ratio of magnesium chloride [http://www.saltworks.us/shop/product.asp?idProduct=8]. That last link is a commercial source of salts which are both a potassium and magnesium supplement. However a little of Dead Sea salt's reputation may be because it also contains bromide, which I believe can mute pain somewhat. Bromide is mildly poisonous and an antidote is iodide. Magnesium chloride as pure analytical grade can probably be acquired inexpensively from a chemical supply house.

FERTILIZER

Potassium is sold for fertilizer under the designation "muriate of potash". I have no reason to suspect that it contains any bad poisons. Ultimately it came from the same original source as sea salt, but was the last to evaporate in ancient inland seas. It is without a doubt the least expensive source of potassium. A bag would probably last a life time or two. I have used it both before and after decanting the sediments it contains for several weeks with no obvious bad effects. It may be a reasonable way to go for people too poor to acquire ORT salts if it were decanted. Decanting may be necessary because its red sediments may be high in iron, which is poisonous in large amounts, especially for people with hemochromatosis. I do not know if it contains mercury.

DE-COTI MARSH'S SALTS

In 1957 de Coti-Marsh of England wrote a book advocating various potassium salts as a treatment for rheumatoid arthritis. He proposed many negative ions to be associated with the potassium. He was the first to definitively propose potassium as an rheumatoid arthritis remedy. The pioneering efforts about potassium for rheumatoid arthritis by Charles de Coti-Marsh enabled him to form a foundation currently active in England that encourages people to use of potassium supplements in order to increase cell potassium and it has helped more than 3500 people cure rheumatoid arthritis [http://www. arthriticassociation.org.uk].

ATHLETIC DRINKS

There are several artificial drinks on the market catering to athletes who exercise in the hot weather. They are in actuality, supplements. All but one of those known to me are really sodium chloride supplements. "Brake-Time" put out by Johnson and Johnson is a sodium supplement, but it also has small amounts of potassium, about equal to the potassium in blood fluids, in addition to vitamin C, phosphate, chloride, and a somewhat lower sugar content than the other athletic fluids. The reason given for lower sugar is to decrease the retention time in the stomach [from Johnson and Johnson brochures]. These drinks are designed to prevent four types of disorders that are associated with heat, as follows:

1. Heat cramps are caused by large sodium chloride losses in sweat. The symptoms are headache, dizziness, fatigue, nausea, vomiting, muscle cramps and circulatory failure in late stages. It can occur from any sweating, even shoveling snow. Muscle cramps are thought to be possible even when cell potassium is low, and may even be more likely then from too high a serum potassium relative to the cell.

2. Water intoxication can occur if a body low in sodium is inundated with pure drinking water. The symptoms are cramps, fever and confusion. The symptoms are similar to alcohol intoxication. You should not suddenly drink enormous amounts of pure water with no salt when very thirsty. Taken to extreme it can even be fatal. It is called hyponatremia.

3. Heat exhaustion is caused by loss of body salts in general, but with strong overtones of potassium loss. Symptoms include muscle weakness, lassitude, nausea, vomiting, and fainting when the body's weight loss is 5% (10% of the water). Treatment can be accomplished with fluids containing sodium and potassium chloride, rest, and cooling. Lane, et al maintains that the minimum daily requirement for potassium on a hot day is over three grams [Lane]. I suspect that it should be considerably higher than that. If a potassium-depleted person who is dehydrated is suddenly supplied with large amounts of pure water, dangerous low blood serum potassium can develop causing respiratory distress [Ellison].

4. Heat stroke is the worst disability because of high death rates. It is a MEDICAL EMERGENCY and is the result of high body temperatures in the vicinity of 105-116 degrees F. The whole heat regulatory mechanism has broken down by this time due partly to damage to brain cells, which damage may be permanent if not corrected immediately. The symptoms are headache, weakness, vertigo (dizziness), and dry skin. Cooling by dousing with water, especially on the head, is imperative. The situation is sufficiently dangerous that medical help should be called immediately, because intravenous fluids may be necessary to prevent death. The body continues to generate heat so time is of the essence so far as cooling the affected person is concerned. Heat stroke is the extreme of heat exhaustion and is also thought to be largely a potassium deficit [Coburn]. Babies can suffer from heat stroke and it is at least as serious to them [http://www.babycenter.com/

refcap/416.html]. Too warm clothes or an overheated car can trigger it. Treatment is the same as adults except it is possible to remove clothing in addition. A potassium deficiency can cause cramps (also called spasms). A potassium deficiency causes severe titanic muscle seizures in chicks [http://jn.nutrition.org/cgi/content/abstract/36/3/351]. Such chicks were near death when those seizures occurred. Some people have what is probably a genetic defect whereby large supplements are required to prevent spasms.

You would think that the athletic drinks fill a real need, at least those containing reasonable amounts of potassium. For the general population they sometimes may if they are available. I address myself to healthy people who presumably are eating a diet that is moderate in sodium and at least adequate in potassium, and reasonably adequate in other nutrients. Such people should rarely be affected by the disorders above if they behave with reasonable common sense. Given that we are discussing such people, water or dilute fruit juice imbibed often in moderate increments should be sufficient and possibly preferable. Vegetable juice is really a food and would probably be inappropriate during strenuous exercise in the absence of a break in the activity.

Paradoxically, low prior sodium intake probably protects people from sodium losses on a hot day. I have no documentation, but I strongly suspect that the time it takes a one gram of sodium per day person is much shorter to become acclimatized than the week or so it is known to take a four gram per day person. The time may be instantaneous or virtually so. I strongly suspect that the high sodium intake of our society is a fair part of the regulatory difficulties of the summer time. A well-fed normal person should be a tough, adaptable person well able to tolerate even fairly unreasonable assaults of temperature and exertion.

In addition to dietary protection against environmental distress, it should be usually possible to solve some of these assaults by planning your activities, by wearing shorts to make use of the considerable heat dissipating area of the legs, using shaded areas, using wide, loose fitting hats, and most effective, dousing with water. Wet clothes would be preferable to damage to your body and brain, and perspiration would probably make you wet anyway. It is possible that moderate perspiration would be advantageous to people whose kidneys have reduced function provided adequate water is available since perspiration glands behave similarly to kidneys.

Therefore I tentatively recommend against drinks high in sodium. It is conceivable that you could get an inadequate sodium intake if you were to happen to select only vegetables low in sodium or only garden vegetables in a low sodium area and at the same time ate no or very small amounts of meat. Such a situation could conceivably introduce dangers. So watch what you eat and consider the possibility of salt supplements, but not necessarily athletic drinks. Salt is much more useful to enhance food flavor than as athletic drinks and in addition is required in at least small amounts to assist in absorbing some of the other nutrients. Also extremely low sodium intakes actually make it more difficult to retain potassium than moderate intakes [Dluhy].

CHAPTER 9
HORMONAL REGULATION OF
POTASSIUM AND SODIUM

SUMMARY

Potassium and sodium are regulated by at least four steroid hormones. ACTH from the pituitary gland in the brain controls these steroids.. Aldosterone is used when potassium intake is high and sodium intake is low. 11-deoxycorticosterone is used when potassium intake is high and sodium intake is high. 18hydroxy-11doxycorticosterone is used when potassium intake is low and sodium intake is low. That last hormone also regulates acidity. 16alpha-18dihydroxy-11deosycorticosterone is used when potassium intake is low and sodium intake is high. Diseases and conditions associated with each of these cases are discussed.

Examination of the results of past experiments on the mineralocorticoid hormones seems to say that they exert their control over kidneys for the purpose of keeping blood serum sodium and potassium content constant by means of at least three and possibly four or more steroid hormones. I believe that aldosterone's role is fairly clear, and well accepted. The others are largely speculations of mine. The three discussed here, besides aldosterone (also called aldocorten, aldocortene, aldocortin, electrocortin, or elektrocortin) are deoxycorticosterone (also called cortexone, 11-desoxycorticosterone, deoxycortone, desoxycortone, compound B, DOCA, or DOC), 18hydroxy-11deoxycorticosterone (also designated 18OH-DOC), and 16-alpha-

18dihydroxy-11deoxycorticosterone which I will designate DOH-DOC. They all must conserve sodium in order to be called a mineralocorticoid.

Sodium makes up most of the cations of blood plasma at 145 milliequivalents per liter (3345 milligrams) where it exceeds potassium 30 times. Potassium makes up most of the cell fluid at about 150 milliequivalents per liter (4800 milligrams)where it exceeds sodium 14 times. Plasma is filtered through the glomerulus of the kidneys in enormous amounts, about 180 liters per day [Potts p261]. Thus 602,000 milligrams of sodium and 33,000 milligrams of potassium are filtered each day. All but the 1000-10,000 milligrams of sodium and the 1000-5000 milligrams of potassium likely to be in the diet must be reabsorbed. Sodium must be reabsorbed in such a way as to keep the blood volume exactly right and the osmotic pressure correct; potassium must be reabsorbed in such a way as to keep serum concentration as close to 4.8 milliequivalents (meq) [Lans] (about 190 milligrams) per liter as possible. Therefore, the sodium kidney's cell wall pumps must always operate to conserve sodium. Potassium must sometimes be conserved also, but because the amount of potassium in the blood plasma is very small and the pool of potassium in the cells is thirty times as large, the situation is not so critical for potassium. Since potassium is moved passively [Bennett] [Solomon] in counter flow to sodium in response to an apparent (but not actual) Donnan equilibrium [Kernan p40, 48] the urine can never sink below the concentration of potassium in serum except sometimes by actively excreting water at the end of the processing. Potassium is secreted twice and reabsorbed three times before the urine reaches the collecting tubules [Wright]. At that point, it usually has about the same concentration as plasma with respect to potassium. If potassium were removed from the diet, there would remain a minimum obligatory kidney excretion of about 200 mg per day when the serum declines to 3.0-3.5 mEq/1 in about one week, [Squires] and can never be cut off completely. Because it cannot be cut off completely, death will result when the whole body potassium declines to the vicinity of one-half full capacity. At the end of the processing, potassium is secreted one more time if the serum potassium is too high.

The potassium moves passively through "gates" (cell wall pores) and probably through one of the cell wall pumps which also pumps sodium, three sodium ions for each two potassium ions. Even so, the net apparent effect is active in the tubules. When ions move through cell wall pumps there is a gate in the pumps on either side of the cell wall and only one gate can be open at once. As a result 100 ions are forced through per second. Pores have only one gate and there one kind of ion only can stream through at 10 million to 100 million ions per second [Gadsby]. For a diagram of how the potassium pores are viewed currently, see Miller's article [Miller]. In order to open the pore requires calcium [Jiang] although it is thought that the calcium works in reverse by blocking at least one of the pores [Shi (has detailed pictures of the atoms in the pump)] Carbonyl groups inside the pore on the amino acids mimics the water hydration that takes place in water solution [Zhou] by the nature of the electrostatic charges on four carbonyl groups inside the pore [Noskov]. You may see a history of the development of the cell wall pump theory in [http://cmbi.bjmu.edu.cn/news/report/2003/nobel2003/ RoderickMacKinnon/15.pdf]. You may see an elaborate discussion of the function of each of the many kidney processes and tubules in [http://ajprenal. physiology.org/content/274/5/F817.full.pdf].

In addition to the kidneys, the gastric glands, salivary glands, colon, perspiration glands, and maybe the red cells are target organs for the mineralocorticoids. These physiological processes are controlled by members of the voltage-gated ion channel protein super family. This protein super family of 143 members is one of the largest groups of signal transduction proteins. Each member of this super family contains a similar pore structure. Eight families are included in this protein super family—voltage-gated sodium, calcium, and potassium channels; calcium-activated potassium channels; cyclic nucleotide–modulated ion channels; transient receptor potential (TRP) channels; inwardly rectifying potassium channels; and two-pore potassium channels. It is not a good idea to put a strain on these complicated pores that could be avoided by proper nutrition. You may see a discussion of electrolyte pores and channels here [http://pcwww.liv.ac.uk/~petesmif/petesmif/ barriers%20pores%20pumps%20and%20gates/index.htm#1].

I believe I now see how the regulation of sodium and potassium is organized by the mineralocorticoids;

CASE #1: Sodium Intake Is Low; Potassium Intake Is High.

Aldosterone has been shown to be the primary steroid used to control the force and direction of the pumps under this circumstance. When potassium in the serum is higher than 4.8 mEq/1, the zona glomerulosa [Brown] of the adrenal jacket secretes more aldosterone [Lans] and potassium is excreted into the end of the tubules and the collecting ducts [Peterson & Wright]. Aldosterone also increases potassium out flow in the last part of the colon only [Fraser 1971] and increases sodium absorption throughout the colon. In the first part of the colon chloride enters with the sodium while in the last part there is only a potassium - sodium exchange [Dolman]. All this was in rats which make poor experimental animals because they do not secrete cortisol as discussed in chapter 12. The amount of aldosterone secreted is a direct function of the serum potassium [Bauer] [Linas] as probably determined by sensors in the carotid artery [Gann , Cruz & Casper], pressure in the carotid artery [Gann, Mills, & Bartter], the inverse of the sodium intake as sensed via osmotic pressure [Schneider], anxiety [Vening], and of the angiotensin II formation [Brown] [Dluhy] [Williams & Dluhy], which last is a peptide hormone for increasing blood pressure by constricting the arteries just ahead of the capillary bed [Haddy]. Angiotensin II is regulated by renin (a peptide hormone) from the kidneys. Either Depletion of potassium [Albrecht] or increase of sodium suppresses aldosterone [Sealed]. If blood pressure has to be increased by constricting capillaries, which is what angiotensin II does, it is an indication that the body needs more sodium in order to expand blood volume or more potassium to strengthen the heart beat. That is undoubtedly the reason why angiotensin is involved in regulating aldosterone and is the core regulation [Williams & Dluhy]. Sodium restriction sensitizes aldosterone to angiotensin, but not 18hydroxy-corticosterone to angiotensin [Fraser 1978, p282]. Angiotensin II acts synergistically with potassium, and the potassium feedback is virtually inoperative when no angiotensin II is present [Pratt]. A portion of the regulation resulting from angiotensin II must take place indirectly from decreased blood flow through the liver due to constriction of capillaries [Messerli, PT]. When the blood flow decreases so does the destruction of aldosterone by liver enzymes. This may be one of the advantages of getting sufficient exercise. However, the primary regulation is acting directly on aldosterone production because angiotensin II acts synergistically with potassium, and the potassium feedback to aldosterone is virtually inoperative when no angiotensin is present [Pratt][Williams & Dluhy]. Such an arrangement tends to be fail safe. If anything happens to send the blood pressure spiraling upward out of control, when angiotensin II drops out in order to correct the situation, it leaves behind a somewhat enhanced potassium serum concentration which also tends to reduce pressure at serum contents of potassium [Haddy] above 4.8 mEq/liter of potassium, and causes sodium to start to decline by the same failure to stimulate aldosterone. For diagrams of this system see [http://pcwww.liv.ac.uk/~petesmif/petesmif/why%20do%20 we%20need%20kidneys/the%20kidney%20and%20homeostasis.htm?../ body].

ACTH, a pituitary peptide, also has some stimulating affect on aldosterone probably by stimulating DOC formation which is a precursor of aldosterone [Brown]. I suspect that this is an adaptation to inversely help protect the body during diarrhea assuming that the primary purpose of ACTH is to inversely mobilize the body's defenses against potassium wasting intestinal disease [Weber 1998] (see chapter 12). Aldosterone is increased by blood loss [Ruch p1099], pregnancy [Farrell], and possibly by other circumstances such as physical exertion, endotoxin shock, and burns [Glas p209]. The aldosterone production is also affected to one extent or another by nervous control which integrates the inverse of carotid artery pressure [Gann, Mills, & Bartter], pain, posture [Farrell], and probably emotion (anxiety, fear, and hostility) [Venning 1956, 1957] (including surgical stress) [Davson p715] [Elman] to produce an unknown messenger hormone which stimulates aldosterone secretion. It is possible that this hormone may now be known and may possibly be thrombin or trypsin [http://joe.endocrinology-journals.org/cgi/reprint/169/3/581.pdf]. Regulation of aldosterone is extremely complicated. I suspect the main reason why emotion is factored in, especially anxiety, is that the aldosterone operates by diffusing to the nucleus to produce a messenger RNA and the various steps take about an hour to come completely on stream [Sharp]. Thus, there is an advantage in an animal anticipating a future need from interaction with a predator because too high a serum content of potassium has very adverse affects on nervous transmission . Anxiety's effect can be discordant. People with an anxiety neurosis can have as high as four times the secretion as normal and people with schizophrenia have a low secretion [Lamson]. This circumstance may be a large part of the affect that placebo manipulation has on experiments. That system has been well studied and its major features are not subject to much doubt. Potassium feedback is the main regulation of aldosterone in normal diet and health, and the other features of aldosterone's regulation are for the purpose of fine tuning and forestalling future circumstances.

The slope of the response of aldosterone to serum potassium is almost independent of sodium intake [Dluhy]. Aldosterone is much increased at low sodium intakes, but the rate of increase of plasma aldosterone as potassium rises in the serum is not much lower at high sodium intakes than it is at low. Feedback by aldosterone concentration itself is of a non morphological character (that is, other than changes in the cells' number or structure) and is poor so the electrolyte feedbacks predominate short term [Glaz]. Thus, the potassium is strongly regulated at all sodium intakes by aldosterone when the supply of potassium is adequate, which it usually is in primitive diets. Aldosterone averages 10 times as high or so among Yanomamo South American Indians as people in our society because their potassium intake averages four times as high and sodium is much lower [Oliver]. On the other hand, if a low potassium diet is fed, the aldosterone declines 5 times in only 24 hours and potassium excretion in the tubules virtually stops in 2 days, by stopping of secretion the first 24 hours and after that by reabsorption caused by low cell content within 72 hours [Linas] The known stimulation by aldosterone of the sodium pump that secretes potassium into the distal loop of the tubules [Stanbury], along with the nature of the potassium feedback already mentioned, make aldosterone certainly a hormone for unloading potassium. As much as 26 grams of potassium can be unloaded per day by healthy people accustomed to a large intake [Peterson CG]. Aldosterone is heavily relied on during high plasma potassium for the aldosterone secretion rises seven fold between 5 milliequivalents and six milliequivalents of potassium in the blood [Braley]. That aldosterone amount makes available the sodium in the bones, which contain nearly half the body's sodium, and is circumstantial evidence that the body depends considerably on aldosterone to keep the serum sodium retained and normal [Davson p717]. Aldosterone keeps the sodium and potassium normal in mononuclear leucocytes [Wheling].

The interrelation of aldosterone with peptide protein hormones is rather complicated. For instance, alpha-melanocyte-stimulating hormone (alpha-MSH) stimulates aldosterone but is itself changed by other peptide proteins [http://www.pubmedcentral.nih.gov/articlerender.fcgi?artid=1136380   ]. Perhaps the reader can untangle these relationships to the end of yielding useful health and nutritional strategies.

CASE #2 Sodium Intake Is High; Potassium Intake Is High.

Such a case would obtain when well fed primitive humans have a clam bake or find a salt lick. It is still necessary to unload potassium, but sodium retention must be less strenuous. I suspect that DOC (deoxycorticosterone) is used for this purpose. DOC stimulates the collecting tubules (the tubules which branch together to feed the bladder) [O'Neil] to continue to excrete potassium in much the same way that aldosterone did but not like aldosterone in the end of the looped tubules (distal) [Peterson & Wright]. At the same time it is not nearly so rigorous at retaining sodium as aldosterone [Ellinghaus], more than 20 times less. DOC accounts for only 1% of the sodium retention normally [Ruch]. In addition to its inherent lack of vigor there is an escape mechanism controlled by an unknown non steroid hormone [Pearce] which overrides DOC's conserving power after a few days just as aldosterone is overridden also [Schacht]. This hormone may be the peptide hormone kallikrein [Majima], which is augmented by DOC and suppressed by aldosterone [Bonner]. If sodium becomes very high, DOC also increases urine flow [O'Neil]. DOC has about 1/20 of the sodium retaining power of aldosterone [Oddie] and is said to be as little as one per cent of aldosterone at high water intakes [Desaulles]. Since DOC has about 1/5 the potassium excreting power of aldosterone [Oddie] it probably must have aldosterone's help if the serum potassium content becomes too high. DOC's injections do not cause much additional potassium excretion when sodium intake is low [Bauer]. This is probably because aldosterone is already stimulating potassium outflow.

When sodium is low DOC probably would not have to be present, but when sodium rises aldosterone declines considerably, and DOC probably tends to take over.

DOC has a similar feedback with respect to potassium as aldosterone. A rise in serum potassium causes a rise in DOC secretion [Brown], which is the correct response for this thesis. However, sodium has little affect [Schambelan & Biglieri], and what affect it does have is direct [Oddie]. Angiotensin (the blood pressure hormone) has little affect on DOC [Brown], but DOC causes a rapid fall in rennin, and therefore angiotensin I, the precursor of angiotensin II [Grekin]. Therefore, DOC must be indirectly inhibiting aldosterone since aldosterone depends on angiotensin II. Sodium, and therefore blood volume, is difficult to regulate internally. That is, when a large dose of sodium threatens the body with high blood pressure, it cannot be resolved by transferring sodium to the intracellular (inside the cell) space. The red cells would have been possible, but that would not have changed the blood volume. Potassium, on the other hand, can be moved into the large intracellular space, and apparently it is by DOC [Grekin] in rabbits since DOC injections lowered serum potassium but did not alter excretion. Thus, a problem in high blood potassium can be resolved somewhat without jettisoning too much of what is sometimes a dangerously scarce mineral and a mineral which reduces the force of the heart during a deficiency. Movement of potassium into the cells would intensify the sodium problem somewhat because when potassium moves into the cell, a somewhat smaller amount of sodium moves out [Rubini]. Thus, it is desirable to resolve the blood pressure problem as much as possible by the fall in rennin above, therefore avoiding loss of sodium, which was usually in very short supply on the African savannas where human ancestors probably evolved.

At the same time dangerous problems with low blood potassium can be avoided somewhat because DOC inhibits glycogen formation [Bartlett], so at low potassium intakes glucose surges are less likely to cause low blood potassium. The resemblance of the pattern of the electromotive forces produced by DOC in the kidney tubules to normal potassium intake, and the total dissimilarity of their shape as produced by potassium deficient tubules, [Helman] would tend to support the above view. The above attributes are consistent with a hormone that is relied upon to tend to unload both sodium and potassium.

DOC's action in augmenting kallikrein, the peptide hormone thought to be the sodium "escape hormone," and aldosterone's action in suppressing [Bonner] [Wright & Davis] it is also supportive of the above concept.

ACTH has more affect on DOC than on aldosterone. I suspect that this is to give the immune system control over electrolyte regulation during diarrhea [Weber 1998] because during the dehydration that diarrhea produces, aldosterone virtually disappears any way [Merrill] even though renin and angiotensin rise high. It is for this loss of aldosterone reason that potassium supplements are very dangerous during dehydration and must not be attempted until at least one hour after rehydration. DOC's primary purpose is to regulate electrolytes. It has other affects on copper enzymes, proteins and connective tissue which I believe is used by the body to help survive during potassium wasting intestinal diseases. Most of the DOC is secreted by the zona fasciculata of the adrenal cortex which also secretes cortisol, and a small amount by the zona glomerulosa which secretes aldosterone.

The greater efficiency of DOC in permitting sodium excretion (or perhaps it should be expressed as inefficiency at retention) must be partly through morphological changes in the kidney cells because escape from DOC sodium retention takes several days to materialize, and when it does, these cells are much more efficient at unloading sodium if sodium is then added than cells accustomed to a prior low intake. Thus, paradoxically, a low salt intake should be protective against loss of sodium in perspiration. Progesterone prevents some of the loss of potassium by DOC [Wambach]. Maybe this is related somehow to the resurgence of rheumatoid arthritis that sometimes happens after pregnancy is over.

CASE #3: Sodium Intake Is Low; Potassium Intake Is Low.

Someone living on the African savanna, profusely perspiring and confined to eating seeds, or worse yet, nothing at all, could find himself in this situation. When potassium becomes low, the first thing that happens is that excretion of potassium from the far end of the kidney tubules and collecting tubules declines. This happens within 24 hours and virtually stops in 2 days. [Bauer]. The large decline in aldosterone secretion [Bauer] is undoubtedly a large part of it. However, it is still necessary to rigorously conserve sodium, and I tentatively propose that this is the function of 18OH-DOC. I have no direct evidence for this yet, but there is strongly suggestive circumstantial evidence. Under low sodium intake 18OH-DOC is increased in serum [Williams, Braley & Underwood]. There is a marked increase in serum 18OH-DOC after injection of insulin [Sparano] [Hiatt] and this may be due to the hypokalemic (low serum potassium) tendency after a rise in insulin [Flatman] which in turn would make the serum more acidic.

18OH-DOC lowers urine pH but has no affect on potassium excretion [Nicholls] [Damasco]. This would seem to indicate that 18OH-DOC's primary purpose is to stimulate hydrogen ion or ammonium excretion. If so, its use by the body to conserve potassium would be indirect by virtue of hydrogen ion's interference with potassium excretion and perhaps strongly dependent on the potassium cell or plasma content, because in potassium deficient rats markedly less 18OH-DOC is converted to 18OH-corticosterone and less yet if sodium is deficient [Muller]. It would also hint that the large affect that ACTH has on 18OH-DOC, causing 18OH-DOC to go down to zero when ACTH does [Tan], revolves primarily around keeping serum immune enzymes at a low pH (high acid) during infection by inhibiting 18OH-DOC's secretion upon declining, and therefore also inhibiting acid excretion. It probably is important normally to keep the vacuoles where pathogens are digested at a high pH because if the pH or alkalinity is not high enough, the pathogens inside the cells are not digested [Ahluwalia]. So when an intestinal or other disease is not calling for ACTH to decline, the potassium conserving attribute of 18OH-DOC by virtue of stimulating acid excretion may be valuable. Perhaps additional experimentation will cast some light on 18OH-DOC.

Insulin is used by the body to counter high serum potassium only at low potassium intakes. At high intakes the affect of insulin stays normal [Knochel]. Thus insulin would help correct surges in serum potassium without the body losing potassium during low intakes. It is possible that the 18OH-DOC does not act directly on electrolytes, but, in addition to the above hydrogen ion affect, through a synergistic or blocking action on other hormones. I suspect that 18OH-DOC acts primarily by blocking aldosterone's affect on potassium, and must have aldosterone to assist it with sodium. Nichols, et al, have been able to show that injection of 18OH-DOC, which raised blood levels of this hormone ten times, were more retentive of sodium than a similar amount of aldosterone. So there must be a synergism involved. At the same time, the ratio of sodium to potassium excretion declined very little for 18 OH-DOC, while for aldosterone, the ratio fell to as little as 1/3 that of control men [Nichols 1966]. This implies a considerable sparing of potassium by 18OH-DOC. If the original aldosterone could have been removed from the serum first, it is possible that the difference would have been greater yet for potassium.

Angiotensin II has very little affect on 18OH-DOC [Melby 1976] and is ambiguous nor does serum potassium above 4.8 meq/litter (187 mg) [Biglieri].- This last is not surprising since 18OH-DOC should not be used by the body at high serum potassium. Under low sodium intake, 18OH-DOC rises in the serum [Williams 1976], which is the correct response for the proposed purpose. ACTH causes a marked increase in 18OH-DOC [Moore] up twenty fold [Melby, Dale & Wilson], probably by a generalized affect on the zona fasciculata of the adrenal cortex where 18OH-DOC is synthesized. I believe that the decline in 18OH-DOC when ACTH declines implied by this is part of the defense against diarrhea already mentioned because of the dehydration that ensues then and thus the need to preserve osmotic pressure by unloading sodium and to some extent potassium. Also it is possible that it is also related to a necessity of immune enzymes to operate more vigorously at higher pH (lower acidity) inside the cell. Large amounts of ACTH have a greater affect on 18OH-DOC than on cortisol [May]. When ACTH drops to zero, 18OH-DOC does also [Tan]. I have not seen evidence so far that cholera enterotoxin, or any other aspect of digestive disease except dehydration [Aguilera] directly affects ACTH yet. If this hypothesis is correct, some other aspect of diarrhea might affect ACTH.

More important to know would be the affect of 18OH-DOC has on angiotensin II because at low serum potassium situations, the intracellular (inside the cells) potassium is usually decreased and this depresses heart contraction strength. I suspect that 18OH-DOC will be found to stimulate angiotensin II rather than the reverse if it has an affect because the intracellular potassium is much more important than serum potassium on the strength of heart contractions [Libretti] [Biglieri]. So when heart contraction strength decreases from low potassium status, it should be imperative to contract the capillaries in order to make sure that blood pressure does not drop. This is likely because the relaxation of capillaries by potassium between 4 and 8 meq/liter serum content is some kind of an adaptive circumstance rather than an inherent characteristic of pre capillary blood vessels. Whether the above stimulation has evolved or not, I don't know since I know of no experimental data.. If this hunch is correct, the low sodium status in this case would reinforce its evolution because low serum sodium's affect on volume also decreases blood pressure. While direct evidence is not available to me, it has been demonstrated that there is more of a marked rise in renin and therefore angiotensin II at low potassium intake than at any other electrolyte status [Douglas]. In any case, 18 OH-DOC is deeply involved in one of the three forms (at least) of high blood pressure (hypertension) [Melby 1972 p323]. However angiotensin II apparently does cause a drop in 18 OH-DOC [Williams 1976] which might be a negative feedback kind of phenomenon, but how it fits into the regulation picture I have not been able to determine.

It is possible that the steroid known as 19-Oxo-deoxycorticosterone is a steroid used by the body to prevent potassium excretion. I believe it would warrant further investigation.

CASE #4: Sodium Is High; Potassium Is Low.

Any of our progenitors who managed to find a salt lick and nothing but seeds, or worse yet, nothing at all, would find themselves in this circumstance. Modern man eating only starchy, salty refined food would also be there.

Someone with diarrhea would probably also be because the dehydration creates a serum artificially high in sodium concentration and because when water can't be absorbed in the lower intestinal tract, potassium can't be either and is lost. For this situation, I propose DOH-DOC (16alpha-18 dihydroxy-deosycorticosterone). DOH-DOC increases the sodium to potassium ratio in urine slightly when injected into rats. This slight increase takes place even when small amounts of aldosterone are injected at the same time. That amount of aldosterone injected alone lowered the ratio slightly [Fuller]. Unfortunately, rats are not good experimental animals for experiments on a hormone possibly used during diarrhea because rats have something in their digestive fluid which neutralizes cholera enterotoxin. [Donowitz]. Also, their ascending colon increases water absorption under c-AMP stimulation, opposite the affect in the descending colon and in other animals [Hornyck]. Thus, the enterotoxin of diarrhea undoubtedly has much less affect on rodents. DOH-DOC combined with aldosterone is more retentive of sodium than aldosterone alone, while DOH-DOC does not retain sodium itself [Melby & Dale 1976] [Dale]. DOH-DOC does not displace aldosterone in general. [Fuller]. DOH-DOC must act in conjunction with aldosterone. If both are secreted together, sodium would be drastically conserved. In other words DOH-DOC acts inversely to unload sodium. If aldosterone drops out, there would be a precipitous loss of sodium retention since DOH-DOC alone has no affect on sodium [Melby & Dale 1976], while at the same time, if my contention is correct, potassium would cease to be excreted in the tubules. I suspect that DOH-DOC has its greatest effect on sodium in the colon because it is here where it would be most advantageous to unload sodium in order to keep water loss in the kidneys at a minimum. I know of no evidence for any colon effect. Its affect on potassium excretion would be most valuable in the kidneys, and this may be why it interferes with DOC's potassium excretion stimulation in the kidneys [Linas]. Conversion of 18OH-DOC to DOH-DOC is greatly increased in the kidneys of low renin patients [Melby & Dale 1977]. Under such a circumstance sodium could be much more strongly retained as long as aldosterone was present and potassium more retained in any case. Not many experiments have been performed on DOH DOC, so more assured conviction that this is the hormone acting inversely for case #4 will have to wait, and there are no experiments I know of to this date.

It may yet be found that angiotensin II or renin do not increase DOH-DOC, but that DOH-DOC decreases angiotensin II in the vicinity of 4.8 meq/liter of potassium and then considerably increases it if the intracellular (cell interior) potassium becomes low. If the mechanism is such that both trends are not possible, then only the second should obtain, for in matters of regulation it is the extreme circumstances which should prevail if a compromise becomes necessary, those circumstances when an animal is fighting for its life.

When DOC is injected into people, it creates malaise, headache, loss of appetite, insomnia and muscle cramps [Relman]. It is possible that some of these symptoms are actually arising from increased internal secretion of DOH-DOC which may be resulting from retention of sodium and loss of potassium implied in the use of DOC injections. It is unlikely that the DOC is causing these symptoms directly because they do not appear when a diet high in sodium and potassium raises DOC in the body. The body may be using DOH-DOC to create some of those symptoms and feelings in order to help to protect it from excessive action during diarrhea. Some of the damaging effects of DOC injections on the heart [Melby, et al 1972] may arise this way also. The loss of appetite, if it exists, would be especially valuable during diarrhea. If DOH-DOC is important during diarrhea as I suspect, it could be that ACTH inhibits it, and thus stimulates it upon ACTH's decline, or at least ACTH has no affect. I know of no information on this.

CONCLUSIONS

By secreting various ratios of the above steroids in conjunction with renin, the angiotensins, ADH water retaining hormone, thirst and unknown supporting hormones, fairly accurate fine tuning should be possible of sodium, potassium, serum volume, osmotic pressure, hydrogen ion, and blood pressure. The cell status is maintained largely by controlling the serum.

I suspect that the distant ancestors of man evolved primarily as fruit, nut and leaf eaters of broad leafed plants, using meat as a fortuitous supplement [http://www.ajcn.org/cgi/content/full/71/3/665?ijkey=XCZg3n3ipAk16]. The tooth design is almost conclusive evidence of a herbivore, the salivary gland which dissolves starch is strongly suggestive of nuts and seeds, and the present day eating preferences of most people is supportive of broad leafed (dicotyledon) plants and seeds. Such a diet is low in sodium and fairly high in potassium [Abernethy]. If so, and I am right about the above, we are organized around aldosterone. I suspect that when we depart from this possibly ideal state for any length of time, we lay ourselves open to the statistical chance of degenerative diseases because our other physiologic processes are geared to this hormone balance.

I suspect that Case #2 may be associated with the form of hypertension which is hard to reverse. The reason I suspect this is that DOC is associated with increased synthesis of collagen and it is possible this tends to increase the thickness of artery walls [Cox] with time and decrease their elasticity. The much greater tendency to grow excess connective tissue when foreign bodies such as silica are imbedded in the skin during DOC injections [Desaulles] [Pospisilova] would give circumstantial support to such an explanation.

Case #3 is probably furnishing some of the symptoms of rheumatoid arthritis because there is a consistently low whole body potassium content in this disease [LaCelle], aldosterone is low in arthritics [Cope], and personal experience is supportive [Weber 1974]. Indicative is that arthritis has been produced by DOC injections [Selye]. I have no information on the status of 18OH-DOC in rheumatoid arthritis. Anyway, it is probable that the bulk of the symptoms manifest themselves through cortisol's status and its response modifying factors because this hormone is reduced in its secretion by the affect of low potassium on the zona fasciculata [Mikosha] and because cortisol removes many of the symptoms of rheumatoid arthritis. The amount of potassium to heal rheumatoid arthritis in adults must usually be 3500 milligrams/day or more because this is the amount which permitted slow improvement of a man across a three month time span [Clark], assuming his sodium intake was normal. Black people average 1500 milligrams/day and white people 2000 milligrams/day in Georgia [Grim] which intake would probably not replenish potassium if diarrhea, vomiting, perspiration, emotional stress or other situations caused a deficiency. There is also circumstantial evidence from nutritional experiments using vegetables [Eppinger]. An unpublished experiment using potassium performed on eight subjects' afflicted with rheumatoid arthritis has revealed beneficial results from potassium supplements [Rudin MV, private communication]. Rastmanesh has performed an experiment testing potassium against rheumatoid arthritis with very encouraging results that increased cortisol [Rastmanesh].

I suspect that most of the people who have rheumatoid arthritis, especially young onset, have had their kidneys damaged by poison or disease in such a way as to make them less efficient at retaining potassium or too efficient at excreting it. I suspect bromine gas as one possibility, for instance, since it probably affected me that way. Some infectious diseases may have a similar effect. An unknown mycoplasma bacteria has been suggested as being involved, and may be the primary cause with potassium deficiency making it impossible for the body to kill the bacteria (see chapter 11). In addition some people's immune system may be more sensitive to a potassium deficiency than others, possibly because of inappropriate secretion of one of the peptide hormones.

Case #4 may prove to be associated with degeneration of heart and kidneys, but based primarily on nutritional statistics. It is also possible that case #4 plays a role in suppressed renin hypertension, since there is increased secretion of DOH-DOC in all cases of that last disease [Melby & Dale 1976]. There is no evidence I know of that the DOH-DOC itself causes the damage.

Drifting back and forth between case #3 and #4 may make one more susceptible to heart attacks and periarteritis nodosa, because arthritics have a low cell content to start with, so that this is superimposed on the harmful effects of high sodium intake, whatever they are, the situation could be much worse than when starting from a well nourished body. The higher death rate in arthritics from heart attacks than others is indicative. It seems that low serum potassium by itself in the absence of diuretics or poor kidney function is not a risk for heart disease [Fang]. The large amounts of vitamin B1 fortified in our society no doubt contributes to the debacle because heart disease from low cell potassium is impossible when vitamin B1 is deficient also [Folis]. When arthritics finally die, the usual terminal events are heart attacks, infections, and ruptured blood vessels [Matsuoka]. We have become so accustomed to these distorted statistics that we fail to perceive their oddity. Indians in El Salvador have a heart disease rate one per cent of ours [World Health Organization]. There is very little chance for such a wide disparity not to have an environmental cause, especially nutritional.

Pregnant women increase their DOC secretion 10 times by the end of the pregnancy [Parker 1980] and have a markedly higher secretion before the onset of menstruation [Parker 1981]. It may be that the larger secretion of progesterone which takes place at these times [Parker 1981] makes necessary the enhanced secretion of DOC by virtue of progesterone's interference with DOC's primary purpose [Gornall]. This erratic secretion may have something to do with the much larger rate of rheumatoid arthritis among women. It is not difficult to envision a problem if such large swings became even a little poorly regulated or had to handle odd electrolyte intakes of sodium and potassium.

While understanding the hormonal basis for electrolyte control will not always have a practical nutritional application, it is nevertheless important that it be well understood. Unless the medical establishment understands the physiological basis for nutritional strategy, it will never accept programs with any ardor based on vague nutritional statistics alone. Also, even if it did, some patients would slip through the cracks as we have seen in the potassium vs. vitamin B-1 interaction. Also, sometimes clinical intervention is essential for genetic or cancer malfunctions of the hormonal systems or to help correct massive assaults of poison or injury. It is well to realize clearly what is happening. The abandonment of aldosterone using DOC instead may not prove logical for all cases, for instance. Excess potassium is the main problem in metabolic shock [Fox], yet previous texts about shock did not even so much as mention potassium, and often do not stress it these days. Our nutritional strategy and even our philosophy of life is entwined with understanding hormones.

CHAPTER 10
POTASSIUM PHYSIOLOGY

SUMMARY

Potassium is essential for nerve transmission and to provide cations for the cell.

Symptoms of a potassium deficiency are shown. These include abnormal thirst, inability of kidneys to concentrate fluid, reduction of muscular strength, and reduction of cell alkalinity, Symptoms of a potassium deficiency that are difficult or impossible to reverse are also shown. These include atrophy of the glomerulosa of the adrenals, scarring of the kidneys, destruction of mitochondria, death of heart cells, and increased mortality from stroke. It is proposed that potassium is important for resisting bacterial disease. Rheumatoid arthritis is proposed to be greatly accentuated by potassium deficiency.

DETERMINATION OF POTASSIUM

Potassium physiology is very complicated because it is the main component of the cations in every cell in the body and is controlled by numerous hormones as you saw in chapter 9. The only way direct determinations of cell potassium can be made is by using a whole body scintillation counter. A scintillation counter is an extremely expensive machine that can count the number of x-rays emerging from the body as a result of the radioactive decay of one of the potassium isotopes, K-40. These machines cost well over $100,000 each. Potassium in the body cells is not often determined for patients because of the enormous cost of the equipment, combined with a blind spot for potassium nutrition among doctors. Other methods for determining cell potassium involve biopsies, balance studies which must be conducted for long periods to get valid results [Lambie], isotope dilution studies which are almost as cumbersome [Jasani] and have difficulties with unreliable erratic diffusion to body components. Welt claims to be able to predict cell potassium from serum potassium if a formula is used which uses other ions, especially hydrogen ions (acid). Welt states that 0.1 pH (hydrogen ion or acidity) unit equals 0.63 millimoles of potassium per liter in the serum [Welt 1958 p217]. I am skeptical that it is always reliable. It is the case, though, that if for some reason the serum is more acid than normal, even small drops in serum potassium indicate significant lowering of cell potassium [Surawicz] [Ono]. However in most cases when cell potassium is low the serum potassium is usually low also [Nickel]. Normal potassium in plasma can be half a milliequivalent lower than serum, but analysis within 30 minutes would prevent it [Bellevue]. In any case it is necessary to use plasma determinations and not serum because serum can give incorrectly high results [Ifudu]. Even with careful determination plasma potassium can be incorrectly high by 0.4 milliequivalents per liter because of potassium losses from platelets after blood is drawn during rheumatoid arthritis [Ifudu]. A method has been developed which promises to be accurate and not too cumbersome. This involves the separation of white blood cells out and their subsequent analysis [Patrick]. So far as I know it is not used much The red blood cells, along with the brain, heart, and liver, have modest losses for several weeks during a deficiency. The muscles suffer most of the losses, possibly due to a reversible 80% decline in pumping sites [Noergaard]. So red cell content can not be used as a criteria. The upshot is that cell potassium is largely invisible to doctors. However, there is an observation of lower potassium in the saliva of rheumatoid arthritis patients [Syrjanen] and often low serum potassium [Cockel], even though the platelets release potassium into the serum when blood is drawn [Ifudu]. There also has been developed recently a method that uses electron bombardment of a single mouth mucous cell by electrons in order to generate distinctive x-rays [http://www.exatest.com/Research.htm]. It is said to cost $175 and determines other electrolytes inside the cell at the same time. This is very encouraging if it proves to be valid. An indication should be possible also by determining what percentage of a potassium supplement is retained by analysis of the daily urine total.

You must be thinking that surely scientists must have created deficiencies of potassium and observed their effects. This is indeed true, at least with animals. Experiments with humans are extremely dangerous because permanent damage can be inflicted on the heart and kidneys [Rubini 1961]. I know of no long term deficiency experiments on people. Rheumatoid arthritis, at least, is difficult to diagnose in animals since they have no way of describing pain, and because there are no sure laboratory tests for rheumatoid arthritis other than low potassium, which we already know is going to be low in a deficiency. Also the most common experimental animals, rodents, do not use cortisol, as will be discussed in chapter 12, and cortisol is deeply involved in rheumatoid arthritis.

SYMPTOMS OF A POTASSIUM DEFICIENCY

Active excretion of potassium virtually ceases in the kidney tubules after two days on a low potassium diet [Linas]. A small part of the potassium that originally entered the kidneys through the glomerulus continues to be excreted, and potassium loss can not be completely cut off. The ability of the kidneys to conserve sodium is impaired. This is because of a decline of aldosterone, no doubt.

Urinary excretion of calcium, magnesium and phosphate is higher during a potassium deficiency in dahl rats. Increasing potassium with potassium carbonate in menopausal women who have low serum potassium results in bone uptake of calcium and phosphorus [http://www.mgwater.com/minbal. shtml], so this circumstance must be similar in humans. It has been proposed that this bone uptake of calcium from increased potassium results partly from salt-induced volume expansion, with an increase in glomerula filtration rate, and partly to competition between sodium and calcium ions in the renal tubule that attends a low calcium intake coupled to a high salt intake [Heany]. Reduced salt or increased calcium makes the potassium reaction disappear. Frassetto, et al, propose that the phenomenon is somehow associated with the acidosis that attends a low potassium intake [Frassetto]. The concept is backed up by epidemiological studies of correlation with urinary potassium in older women [Zhui].

It is thought that the reduction of magnesium is what causes the association of potassium with hypertension by virtue of the affect of magnesium on the power of the potassium-sodium cell wall pumps. Six months are required of magnesium supplements before complete normalization of pumps [Dorup]. You may see a long list of articles on the above subjects here [http://www.lef. org/prod_hp/abstracts/potassiumabs.html].

The fluid inside the cells shows a decrease in potassium, alkalinity, and phosphate [Gardner 1953] but no reduction of potassium in rat brain and liver, 18% in heart and kidneys, and 48% in muscle [Southon]. Part of the lost potassium inside the cells is replaced by sodium [Rubini 1972]. This is probably the reason why there is increased edema when potassium is repleted at first [Welt 1960 p245] because the sodium is forced out of the cells then. Arginine [Iacobellis] and lysine [Eckel], which are amino acids having a positive charge, show a marked rise in the fluid of some cells in some animals, going from almost zero to 8% of the positive ions. Adequate potassium has been shown to be necessary for protein synthesis [Cannon 1951]. There is considerably less protein metabolized in deficient chicks [Rinehart]. The positive ions, calcium and magnesium, increase inside the cells and the cell becomes more acidic [Gardner 1950]. If these are adaptations to solve a potassium deficiency, such elaborate mechanisms are an indication that potassium is much more of a problem in nature than medical people think, let alone in our potassium-starved society. The diarrhea diseases are the primary problem for this in nature, no doubt. DNA synthesis inside the muscle cell is decreased during a deficiency [Truong]. Failure to maintain sufficient potassium in the cells, results in the accumulation of sodium, waste products, toxins, calcium and acid in the cell. Eventually cells can become inefficient or fail to function entirely.

An abnormal thirst is also thought to be frequently present in a potassium deficiency. Increased water intake rises to a peak in dogs in 3 to 7 weeks, then declines to normal [Smith].

Perhaps it would be a good idea to determine as many of these circumstances as are possible without a biopsy while people are healthy so that when they become sick the potassium status can be easily estimated without expensive machinery or long time delays.

I can not be certain that all the phenomena above are caused by an acute deficiency in humans, but most are quickly and easily reversible in animals. Most of the data that do not require analysis of internal organs have been confirmed in humans.

Effects that are not easily reversible or involve structural changes in the body's cells are as follows:

The part of the adrenal gland (zona glomerulosa) which synthesizes aldosterone atrophies [Cope p432]. Fat (they probably meant cholesterol) is deposited in the vascular system. This deposition is probably reversible [Davis] [Strauss]. More serious is lesions of the kidneys in hypertensive salt loaded rats and permanent scarring of the kidneys which is probably irreversible [Holman]. Welt believes that the consensus is that kidney damage is reversible, however, and is largely in the distal tubules and collecting ducts [Epstein p272] with no visible changes in the glomeruli [Welt 1960 p224,225]. Calcification is prominent during phosphate loading [Welt 1960 p225]. Small particles in the cell called ribosomes have the internal structure lastingly altered. Mitochondria of the collecting tubules swell and disrupt [Kark]. Certain cells in the kidneys that have a darker color than the others increase in numbers. There are also abnormalities in the structure of other kidney cells [Rhodin] [Naslund][Strauss]. Cells in the lining of the tubules are most affected in dogs

[Tate]. The above is based on animal experiments. Man rarely has kidney destruction that appears the same as the rat's or dog's. Localized death of heart cells is usually found in the species observed [Rowinski][Folis][Molnar] but is not always observed in every individual [Tate]. Heart lesions from a potassium deficiency are well established. The fibers lose striations and assume a hyaline appearance [Folis 1953]. This depends on an adequate sodium intake [Cannon 1953]. However because sodium is almost always accompanied by chloride, I am not sure that this relationship is accurately known yet since it could be the chloride which is giving part or even all of the problem. Heart disease is discussed in chapter 3 and will also be discussed at greater length in the potassium supplement chapter 8.

There is a striking, consistent alteration of the kidneys' ability to concentrate fluids in humans. This impairment reverses in one and a half to four years after relieving a deficiency, but not always [Hollander p933]. I suspect that this is to maintain urine flow by excreting water in order to reduce potassium loss that would otherwise obtain if the urine had a potassium concentration the same as serum.

Potassium is thought to be essential to defense against pathologic bacteria on the basis of increased liability to infection in deficient kidneys [Woods] that have suffered no change otherwise. It may be that the reason for this has been found. It seems that the white cell vacuole requires an alkaline medium in order to both kill and digest microbes. To achieve this it must pump potassium into the vacuole using a calcium activated (Bkca) pump. This is known because, when a chemical blocks this pump channel, microbes are not killed in spite of normal phagocytosis (engulfing of microbes) and oxidase activity [Ahluwalia]. So it seems plausible to me that, when the pump is operating normally in the absence of the above poison, a low cell potassium would make it more difficult to achieve the enhanced alkalinity. This may be the reason why potassium deficient kidneys are susceptible to infection and other infections may yet prove to be overcome with more difficulty, possibly even mycobacteria. If mycobacteria are causing rheumatoid arthritis as some suspect, this could explain why potassium supplements cures rheumatoid arthritis.

Muscular strength is directly related to potassium intake [Judge]. Paralytic blockage of the lower intestines, which sometimes attends surgery, is probably contributed to by low potassium [Lowman]. Rats have symptoms during a deficiency that include abdominal distention, lethargy, sagging organs, and loss of tone, and sometimes decreased movement of the intestines [Schrader]. A potassium deficiency seems to be most destructive to the tissues that derive from the middle layer of the embryo, mesenchyme tissue [Seekles]. These tissues include all the connecting tissues, the heart, the blood vessels, the kidneys and the white blood cells. A potassium deficiency causes a higher mortality during stroke. This increase is independent of age, severity of the stroke, blood pressure, history of hypertension, or smoking [Ganballa, et al].

CONCLUSIONS

I can not be certain that all the phenomena above are caused by an acute deficiency in humans, but most are quickly and easily reversible in animals. Most of the data that do not require analysis of internal organs have been confirmed in humans.

I have not been able to find out which hormones regulate chloride excretion, if any.

Perhaps it would be a good idea to determine as many of these circumstances as are possible without a biopsy while people are healthy so that when they become sick the potassium status can be easily estimated without expensive machinery or long time delays.

In any case, getting enough potassium from food is a much superior strategy for protecting potassium than degrading glutamine to ammonium. Glutamine is used as a nitrogen shuttle during infection [Labow], and preventing glutamine loss may be part of the protection by potassium against infection. Fortunately getting enough potassium in food is not nearly as complicated as what happens to it after it arrives in the body.

Potassium physiology is indeed, complicated. But you do not have to be on top of all of that. All you have to do is as follows;

1. Eat only unprocessed food.

2. Do not burn or boil it, or if you boil it, drink the boil water.

3.   Do not add any poison to it, such as aspartame, aluminum, fluoride, etc.

4. Do not eat, drink, or breathe any poison between meals.

5. Do not allow yourself to become thirsty.

6. Eat a little meat, milk, or eggs at every meal.

7. Get out in the sun or take vitamin D tablets.

8.   Take iodide supplements and maybe selenium and vitamin C also.

If people were to do all of that, a large majority of people will live long, healthy lives.

CHAPTER 11
HISTORY OF RHEUMATOID
ARTHRITIS RESEARCH

SUMMARY

Research on rheumatoid arthritis in the past has been performed as spurred by several hypotheses. These were; stress hormones, copper or boron deficiency, bacterial infection with mycobacteria, mycoplasmin, or amoebas, .a hypothesis that the body's own immune system attacks the joints for some mysterious reason, that Epstein barr virus is involved, some kind of allergy, poisons in nightshade related foods or something added to coffee, and poisons such as fluoride in drinking water. Of course you already know of my efforts to relate a potassium deficiency to rheumatoid arthritis. Medicines have been developed, but they are largely palliative.

For years rheumatoid arthritis was the poor relation of medical research. Its victims did not do something dramatic like quickly die, as they often did with pneumonia, or go insane as they did with syphilis, or bring tears to the eyes as with childhood diphtheria, or have nice bright, easily recognizable symptoms as with measles. Rheumatoid arthritis tended to be a disability of old folks with vague, sometimes disbelieved symptoms. That has changed and extensive, well-funded research is being done now partly because there has been a considerable increase in rheumatoid arthritis. Indeed, the Center for Disease Control has said that it is a leading cause of disability in the USA today. Rheumatoid arthritis was first proposed as a separate syndrome by Heberden and Haygarth in the early 19th century. Forming the backdrop of later research are several hypotheses, some borrowed from research into other diseases, and some with a novel twist of their own.

STRESS HORMONES

One of the oldest of these is the stress hormone hypothesis championed by Selye [Selye 1949 & 1950 p197-198]. Roughly his contention was that hormones released by the body, especially those released by the jacket of the adrenal glands, cause an adverse reaction to the joint tissues when they are released in too large amounts or the wrong ratios under conditions of environmental stress or psychic stress. His concept was generalized and only mentioned rheumatoid arthritis as an unlikely possibility. The theory had some plausibility since arthritis can be produced by injecting deoxycorticosterone (DOC), which is a potassium excreting hormone, into a person who has been suffering from Addisons's disease or into animals [Selye et al 1944] [Turner]. Some support is given to this approach in that repressed hostility is probably correlated with rheumatoid arthritis [Cobb]. The dramatic affect that cortisone has on rheumatoid arthritis, removing all symptoms in a short time, would give encouragement to a scientist trying to approach this matter from Selye's viewpoint.Cortisone was first synthesized by Julian, which dramatically lowered its price, and used against rheumatoid arthritis by Kendall and Hench in 1948, This hypothesis has never been refuted although it has fallen into disfavor recently. This is probably because some rather severe side effects materialized eventually when medical people used cortisone for a long time. As one author put it "It is remarkable how cortisone can get a seemingly hopeless patient on his feet again. Sometimes it is so effective that he can walk all the way to the autopsy table."   Cortisone changes to cortisol, which reduces resistance to infection (glucocorticoids, of which cortisol is a member, cause 5 times more likelihood of tuberculosis [Jick]) , suppresses fever, causes polyarteritis nodosa (a blood vessel disease), and suppresses collagen synthesis. Some additional evidence that hormones play a crucial role is that dehydroepiandrosterone (DHEAS] is reduced during inflammatory arthritis [Dessein]. Stress theories did not always emphasize steroid hormones. Histamine was suggested as possibly being involved [Eyring].

A group called "Arthritis Medical Information Society" had revived this concept. They had claimed cures using a "balanced" regime of injected hormones, hormones which include the steroid testosterone, a sex hormone. They claimed a preponderance of anabolic (tissue building) hormones prevent side effects. They also recommend better nutrition, which I suspect, was having the major affect, especially potassium nutrition.

NUTRIENT DEFICIENCIES

Rheumatologists regard any hint that nutrition could have any affect on rheumatoid arthritis as quack medicine and will have nothing to do with it.

McCord has proposed that rheumatoid arthritis may be caused by insufficient amounts of superoxide dismutase, an enzyme catalyzed by copper [McCord]. Copper supplements, either as pharmaceuticals [Sorenson 1980] or as copper bracelets, have been proposed with encouraging results. Copper as ceruloplasmin is high in the blood of rheumatoid arthritics [Zoli] [Louro] and this may be depleting copper by greater excretion through the bile. The reason why copper seemed to impact rheumatoid arthritis may be because a copper deficiency increases mast cells half again as much in rats [Schuschke], which increased numbers in turn increases inflammation caused by histamine release by those mast cells as stimulated by the immune peptide hormones. Also copper is crucial for the immune system, so a mycoplasmin infection to be mentioned later may, for all we know, be more successfully resisted with adequate copper.

A boron deficiency has been proposed as accentuating rheumatoid arthritis. It has been proposed that the high incidence of rheumatoid arthritis in Jamaica and northern Thailand is because of low boron. If so, I have no information as to a possible mechanism.

MICROORGANISMS

Because of the dramatic successes that scientists had in their battle against bacteria and virus, it is not surprising that these men should turn their attention to finding an organism, which was responsible for arthritis. The fact that some infections could trigger an attack of arthritis must have given them encouragement. Therefore, and not surprisingly, infections have been searched for as causal to rheumatoid arthritis. I know of no infection that has been proven to chronically inhabit the joints, although viruses such as parvovirus, chronic hepatitis B virus and hepatitis C have been found to trigger arthritis [Siegel], Lyme disease has been proposed by Malawista, and mycoplasma bacteria have been found to inhabit the synovial fluid [Schaeverbeke] (which is the fluid in the joints) and the joints [Poehlmann p353]. Mycoplasma has produced experimental rheumatoid arthritis in animals [Poehlmann p354].

The mycobacterium, Staphylococcus aureus, produces a persistant septic arthritis [Go]. Mycobacteria are rod-shaped, Gram-positive aerobes, or facultative anaerobes. As deduced from its genome, M. tuberculosis has the potential to manufacture all of the machinery necessary to synthesize all of its essential vitamins, amino acids, and enzyme co-factors. Rashid and Ebringer claim that there are antibodies against Proteus mirabilis in arthritics. They say there is a molecular similarity between "LRREI" amino acid sequences present in small or peripheral joints and "IRRET" motif in Proteus urease enzyme, and this may be why small joints are affected [Rashid]. Wilson, et al, propose that ciprofloxacin, norfloxacin, trimethoprin and sulfamethoxazole will cure Proteus especially with increased fluid and cranberry juice [Wilson]. Ebringer proposes that smoking makes one more susceptible to Proteus [Gorman]. Other infections are known to trigger arthritis and tooth abscesses can cause shoulder bursitis.

Wyburn-Mason suggested that maybe an amoeba causes rheumatoid arthritis [Wyburn-Mason].

Antibiotics ((tetracyclines such as tetracycline, oxytetracycline, doxycycline, especially minocycline, trade named Minocin by Lederle) has been said to be shown to cure many arthritics [Cole]. Those antibiotics are specific against an odd bacterium species devoid of cell walls, which can enter the cells like viruses, called "Mycoplasma". Mycoplasma are flask-shaped and are most likely descended from gram-positive bacteria. They are not the same as mycobacteria. Due to their seriously degraded genome they cannot perform many metabolic functions, such as cell wall production or synthesis of purines. They are believed to contain the absolute minimum machinery necessary for survival. The Mycoplasma cell is built of a minimum set of organelles, including a plasma membrane, ribosomes, and a highly coiled circular chromosome. However the above antibiotics are said to be only maximally affective if the patients stop eating sugars, fats, and grains [Poehlmann]. This would greatly increase potassium intake. High doses have been found to be more effective than low [Kloppenberg]. A clinical trial has shown that 80% of patients show a marked improvement using minocycline [Donta]. You may see a long list of references about the use of minocycline here [http://www.rheumatic.org/studies.htm].

When mycoplasma bacteria are involved, it takes a long time for doxycycline to have an effect. It is said that that medicine has anti-inflammatory affects also, so one can not draw certain conclusions yet. As already mentioned, doxycycline may cause greater magnesium excretion, so supplements of magnesium might be necessary with this medicine. Long time use also creates nausea and photo sensitivity [Donta]. You may see numerous references here [http://www. rheumatic.org/studies.htm]. Tetracycline combined with clindamycin gave significant improvement to 90% of patients in an experiment [Gompel]. Mycoplasmin bacteria as a factor in joint pain is plausible and maybe other pain as well because those bacteria may well be increasing secretion of glucosteroid response modifying factors, although I have no evidence. People low in interferon-gamma are susceptible to mycobacteria and benefit from interferon-gamma treatment [Casanova]. Rothschild believes rheumatoid arthritis first started among Tennessee Indians 4000 years ago and spread from there [http://mcclungmuseum.utk.edu/research/renotes/rn-5txt.htm]. If so, this would be evidence for a bacterial or viral underlying cause.

It is possible that the vitamin D is having a direct affect on rheumatoid arthritis if arthritis is indeed an infection, for it has been discovered that vitamin D activates a cell receptor that activates antimicrobial peptide (cathelicidin), which is involved in killing of bacteria such as tuberculosis bacteria [Liu]. Equally likely would be vitamin D's role in accentuating magnesium absorption, and thus potassium absorption.

When resisting diseases, especially bacterial, there is probably another reason for keeping the cell potassium normal with adequate nutrition. The effectiveness of potassium against rheumatoid arthritis could conceivably be partly due to the ability of a potassium replete body to resist bacterial infection. Potassium is thought to be essential to defense against pathologic bacteria on the basis of increased liability to infection of deficient kidneys [Woods][Kahn] that have suffered no change otherwise, although rat kidneys are not depleted of potassium [Welt 1960, p223]. It may be that the reason for this has been found. It seems that the white cell vacuole requires an alkaline medium in order to both kill and digest microbes. To achieve this it must pump potassium into the vacuole using a calcium activated (Bkca) pump. This is known because, when a chemical blocks this pump channel, microbes are not killed in spite of normal phagocytosis (engulfing of microbes) and oxidase activity [Ahluwalia]. So it seems plausible to me that, even when the pump is operating normally, a low cell potassium would make it more difficult to achieve the enhanced alkalinity. pH inside the cell goes from 6.98 to 6.48 (almost neutral to slightly acid) from potassium depletion (based on assumptions) [Welt 1960, p219] [Gardner]. This may be the reason why potassium deficient kidneys are susceptible to infection and other infections may yet prove to be overcome with more difficulty. I know of no experimental information for the affect on mycoplasma bacteria though, except that rheumatoid arthritis patients are nine times as likely to get tuberculosis, a mycobacteria, than healthy people [Seong].

It is possible that any strategy against mycobacteria would be enhanced if an intracellular enzyme called interferon-ϒ-inducible p47 GTPase (IGTP) in mice that is thought to disrupt a protective membrane around mycobacteria, and thus enable a lysosome sac to destroy the bacteria, could be stimulated. Interferon gamma stimulates the overall process of mycobacteria destruction, but not directly the enzyme itself in humans [Singh]. For this last circumstance I would assume that potassium would be especially effective if the above potassium proposal is valid.

There is a different bacteria called mycoplasmin which has also been

implicated in rheumatoid arthritis according to this site [http://www.
thearthritiscenter.com/arthritis_info.htm#Anchor-Reactive-49575] and
this reference [Ramirez]. 50% of rheumatoid arthritis patients have had
mycoplasmal bacterial infections [Nicolson]. Since mycobacteria are thought
to be possible ancestors of gram positive bacteria [http://users.rcn.com/
jkimball.ma.ultranet/BiologyPages/E/Eubacteria.html] it may yet prove
possible to kill them with anacardic acids in raw cashew nuts as gram positive
tooth infection bacteria are killed [Weber 2005]. Thus also acne, leprosy, and
tuberculosis may also be cured that way. Someone should try it. It should be
tried on mycoplasma as well.

Also it has been proposed that gallium can kill mycobacteria possibly by
interfering with their iron metabolism [Olakanmi]. So maybe it would improve
rheumatoid arthritis, There are cases of people cured of rheumatoid arthritis
by gallium [Olakanmi]. Gallium is an element and cannot be degraded by the
body's enzymes. Therefore experiments with it are inherently dangerous.

Dr. Mirkin has posted instructions for using antibiotics against rheumatoid
arthritis [http://www.drmirkin.com/joints/J106.htm]. It could be that using
all these medicines simultaneously may prove to be especially advantageous.
Do not try it yourself, though, because it could also prove to be dangerous.
It is not likely that pharmaceutical companies will try it since non are able to
be patented. It will have to be a university.

An opioid antagonist drug called Naltrexone (Naltrexone in the large
50mg size, originally manufactured by DuPont under the brand name ReVia,
is now sold by Mallinckrodt as Depade and by Barr Laboratories under the
generic name naltrexone) that blocks some endorphin receptors [http://www.
lowdosenaltrexone.org/index.htm#What is low dose naltrexone]. Said
blockage is thought to cause the body to temporarily secrete more endorphins,
especially after midnight at night. These endorphins are thought to stimulate
the immune system by decreased interleukin-4 and with increased gamma
interferon and interleukin-2 [Sacerdote].

It appears to be especially effective for minimizing symptoms and retarding
progression of multiple sclerosis (MS) [http://www.lowdosenaltrexone.org/
ldn_and_ai.htm] [http://www.lowdosenaltrexone.org/ldn_and_ms.htm
]. There are drugs listed in this site that should not be taken with low
dose Naltrexone, including cortisol [http://www.webspawner.com/users/
avoidthesedrugsonldn/index.html]. There is information in this site for
mitigating side effects, including starting with one milligram doses [http://
www.webspawner.com/users/sideeffectsofldn/index.html]. Advice how
to proceed if you have been taking cortisol may be seen here [http://ldn.
proboards.com/index.cgi?board=links&action=display&thread=773]. Also
see this site for a discussion group [http://www.ldninfo.org]. Low doses

of Naltrexone (LDN), 1.5 to 4.5 milligrams, at bedtime is used (timing is important, and it is important not to buy slow release forms). It is said to have no known bad side effects at those doses [http://www.lowdosenaltrexone.org/index.htm#What_is_low_dose_naltrexone] other than insomnia or stiffness the first week or two in some people.

I think some clinical studies on Naltrexone are in order, and it should not be a prescription drug due to the absence of bad side effects. Though side effects appear unlikely, it is not proven over longer periods. You may see how to obtain Naltrexone without a prescription here [http://www.webspawner. com/users/howtoobtainldn/index.html]

Olive leaf extract has shown clinical evidence of effectiveness against a wide range of viruses, including AIDS [Bihari], herpes, and cold viruses. It sometimes produces a Herxheimer or pathogen die off symptoms (from effectiveness against bacteria?). There is evidence that it is synergistic (mutual enhancement) with Naltrexone. There have been a few case histories of improvement in what were probably rheumatoid arthritis patients. The active ingredient is said to be oleuropein or enolate [http://users.rcn.com/wussery/olive1.html]. There has been very little follow up research done on it.

Also a recent blood analysis has disclosed that rheumatoid arthritis patients have ten times as many Epstein Barr (mononucleosis, herpes) virus antibodies as normal people [Balandraud]. So it is possible that some arthritis is a reaction to antibodies of that virus as the authors suggest. It has been proposed that maybe the inflammation of rheumatoid arthritis arises from a latent herpes virus and that lysine supplements will put it into remission, based on a single case history. It is quite possible that rheumatoid arthritis is triggered by more than one species of pathogen.

It is possible for joints to become directly infected by pathogens, but the symptoms of this fairly rare condition are not exactly the same as rheumatoid arthritis. It causes skin rash, large lymph nodes, fever, and often affects the kidneys and heart However an exhaustive search by me has not disclosed any microbe consistently present in inflamed tissue during rheumatoid arthritis prior to 1975 [Phillips] although some investigators believe that an amebic infection is involved as mentioned above. Nor have I seen anything since. The Arthritis Trust of America and Canada [http://www.arthritistrust.org] is organized around the concept that killing an unknown microorganism with antibiotics will alleviate rheumatoid arthritis and claim to have had some good results. Also research has implicated bacteria called chlamydia in a disease called "reactive arthritis" [Gerard] which usually afflicts a few joints in the knees, ankles, or toes a few weeks or months after infection. When it affects other tissue it is called "Reiter's syndrome" [http://www.drmirkin. com/joints/9094.html]

Antibiotics have been used successfully against sarcoidosis [http://yarcrip. com/sarcoidosissuccumbs-preprint.htm] [Marshall]. Probably sunlight and vitamin D supplements should be avoided during sarcoidosis. Those authors believe that a mycoplasmin like bacteria is responsible for that disease, and suggest that similar bacteria may be involved in rheumatoid arthritis and other diseases like it by infecting white blood cells and causing autoimmunity. So it is also possible that the vitamin D is having a direct affect on rheumatoid arthritis if rheumatoid arthritis is indeed an intracellular infection, for it has been discovered that vitamin D activates a cell receptor that activates antimicrobial peptide (cathelicidin) as mentioned above, which is involved in killing of intracellular bacteria such as tuberculosis bacteria [Liu]. Even more likely would be vitamin D's role in accentuating magnesium absorption, and thus potassium.

AUTOIMMUNE HYPOTHESES

The most popular current hypothesis is the autoimmune hypothesis [http:// www.ucl.ac.uk/~regfjxe/T.htm]. This hypothesis proposes that the body's mechanism for killing disease organisms gets out of order, and starts killing connective tissue cells or perhaps dissolving the connecting tissue itself. No mechanism has been advanced for the immune system getting out of order though. Moderately high statistical associations between rheumatoid arthritis and physiological circumstances that are closely related to the immune system have given investigators all over the world encouragement. Many do not even regard the concept as a hypothesis, but as a proven theory. A much higher association of antigen HLA-B27, which is a known immunity factor, with diseases in the arthritic group such as Reiter's syndrome and ankylosing spondilitis [Mikkelsen] has tended to reinforce this feeling that they are on the right track. Investigations into the autoimmune hypothesis are well funded. A number of medicines have come into use, most of which affect the immune system [http://sock19.tripod.com/socksrheumatoidarthritislinks/id19.html], but usually with bad side effects. These so called NSAIDs (non steroid anti inflammatory drugs) cause quite distinct and severe biochemical damage during drug absorption (uncoupling of mitochondrial oxidative phosphorylation proving to be most important) which results in increased intestinal permeability. All commonly used NSAIDs, apart from aspirin and nabumetone, are associated with increased intestinal permeability in man. Whilst reversible in the short term, it may take months to improve following prolonged NSAID use [Bjarnason].

It would seem strange that mesenchyme tissue (tissue derived from the middle layer of the embryo) is primarily affected, that it would take so long to be destroyed, or that there would be spontaneous remissions if the auto immune hypothesis were valid. At the very least some auxiliary hypotheses would be necessary. Millman has proposed that some of the cell wall of bacterial invaders erode off and become incorporated into the collagen [Millman]. How cell walls would know enough to incorporate symmetrically on either side of the body would be mysterious. Effects of steroid treatment may be due to inhibition of arachidonic metabolic cascade (the prostaglandin hormones) especially to leucotrienes, which are thought to activate macro white cells [Nalbandian]. The hypothesis seems plausible but attempts to adapt it to diagnostic techniques have been unsuccessful. There have been no cures. There have been medicines proposed which dampen the immune system, but most of them cause the joint damage to get worse in the long run and are very dangerous during a different infection.

Currently there is considerable effort being put into exploring the role of the increase in tumor necrosis factor (TNF or cachectin or cachexin) during rheumatoid arthritis. TNF is a peptide protein hormone secreted by the immune system. Encouraging results are obtained by blocking agents [Campbell] such as Remicade, but dampen the immune system. However, that therapy makes the patient more susceptible to infections such as tuberculosis and, if rheumatoid arthritis proves to be a bacterial infection, possibly makes rheumatoid arthritis worse also. It probably receives some of its affect by sensitizing the pituitary gland to secrete more ACTH and therefore stimulating the adrenals to secrete more cortisol [Staub] and thus be nothing more than a palliative affect. It has been proposed recently that GIK (glucose insulin potassium) solutions be used to suppress tumor necrosis factor [Das]. GIK is really an injection of a potassium supplement, with glucose to accompany it into the cells, assisted by insulin. Probably what happens during potassium deficiency is that the low potassium causes cortisol to decline [Mikosha]. This in turn causes superoxide dismutase (an enzyme which degrades extremely active oxides like hydrogen peroxide and superoxide radical) to decline. As a result some of the cells are killed. At the same time the enzyme which cross-links connective tissue, lysil oxidase, is inhibited and this causes severe problems with strength of blood vessels, spinal discs, and even the joints if continued a long time. So GIK solutions would presumably reverse those affects.

There is a hypothesis that the enzymes inside the lysosome sacs inside the white cells are released because of weakness [Weissman]. This may be happening when sodium urate crystals are ingested by the white cells in gouty arthritis or at least pseudogout [Wallingford] but evidence for it in rheumatoid arthritis is inconclusive. In any case the immune system is very complicated. It is too bad that such complicated and expensive autoimmune research is being performed because of what is probably primarily a potassium deficiency's affect on the immune system.

ALLERGY

The hypothesis that rheumatoid arthritis is an allergy is in the same general category as the autoimmune hypothesis. Such a hypothesis has the advantage, not shared by the autoimmune hypothesis directly, of advancing an environmental factor, which is almost certainly involved. The wide geographical variations already mentioned in chapter 3 virtually ensures this. Turnbull has had impressive percentages (50%) of arthritics improved by removing certain foods from the diet [Turnbull]. Others claim success by removing environmental poisons such as cooking gas [Randolph]. Mcdougall had published references to research around allergy affecting rheumatoid arthritis [http://www.drmcdougall.com/newsletter/may_june2.html]. However the diet he recommends is high in vegetables and therefore potassium and magnesium. Medical people do not pay much attention to this allergy hypothesis even as a diagnostic approach. The references on allergy often mention this, and it appears to be true of most of the literature. Zussman, who improved four arthritics this way, could not believe he was dealing with rheumatoid arthritis or was afraid of ridicule, and so entitled his article "Food hypersensitivity simulating rheumatoid arthritis" [Zussman]. Allergens in food are Dong's hypothesis [Dong], but he has no controlled experiments to verify his contention other than the general population being a control.

Allergy is without a doubt part of the rheumatoid arthritis picture since arthritics have two to three times as much incidence of allergy as average [Zeller]. White cells respond to a human nuclei challenge with 3.5 times as much histamine production in arthritics as normal people [Permin]. At one time a hornet's sting caused me to break out in a rash and swell up tremendously. More recently numerous stings from wasps, yellow jackets, and a hornet caused nothing but a sharp moderate pain and irritation for a day or two resembling a mosquito bite. A genetic defect making me incompatible with hornets would surely still be with me. I put bicarbonate of soda (baking soda) on the sting immediately now, but not always and anyway it does not seem possible that this alkalinity would have an affect on an allergic response remote from the wound. This allergic attack preceded my bout with what was probably rheumatoid arthritis at about 50 years of age, which I was able to remove with potassium supplements.

POISON IN FOOD

Similar in practical application to the food allergic hypothesis, but probably physiologically different if valid, is a hypothesis put forward by Childers. He maintains that poisons in the solanaceous family are causing rheumatoid arthritis [Childers]. This is the night shade family and includes tomatoes, potatoes, pepper, eggplant, and tobacco. He suspects a steroid chemical similar to vitamin D in its structure, or possibly one of the solanine alkaloids. If this hypothesis proves valid, it is possible that a substance similar to deoxycorticosterone (DOC) contained in these plants will be found to be responsible [Childers] since deoxycorticosterone stimulates potassium excretion. It is not likely that these foods will have more than an insignificant affect on those eating sufficient potassium if this is the cause of the affect.

A poison that interferes with copper metabolism is another possibility. Smoking tobacco is known to cause emphysema, which is in turn is known to be often caused by a copper deficiency. Childers has had 70% of his volunteers report improvement by deleting these vegetables. However, only 30% responded to his survey [Childers, private communication] so that 70% figure could be as low as 25% or so. Unless rheumatoid arthritis has more than one cause or is misdiagnosed, even 70% is too low to establish anything as a primary cause. While the causal evidence is not excellent, the evidence is suggestive enough to persuade one to remove those vegetables from one's diet while symptoms of rheumatoid arthritis are still present, just in case. There are plenty of other vegetables. Also never eat green or sprouting potatoes raw. Green potatoes have a very virulent poison, virulent enough to kill some people. The poison is destroyed by frying and baking but not by boiling. Also useful to know is that most of the solanines are close to the skin and possibly the other poisons as well [Childers, inside addenda].

Those poisons are not the only ones that can cause, accentuate, or mimic rheumatoid arthritis if indeed they do. Fluoride has been shown to cause joint pains that mimic or are identical with rheumatoid arthritis [http://www.fluoridealert.org/health/bone/fluorosis/arthritis/rheumatoid-arthritis.html]. This is important since many USA municipal water supplies (but not continental Europe) are fluoridated and fluoride insecticides are put on some foods. Fluoride in city water will cause fluorosis discoloration of teeth, weakened bones, damage to the kidneys an immune system, and, worst of all, damage to the nerves resembling Alzheimer's disease. So fluoride water should not be drunk or bathed in regardless of whether one has any kind of arthritis or not.

A recent study has indicated that something in decaffeinated coffee significantly increases the risk of rheumatoid arthritis in women drinking more than 3 cups per day. It is probably residual solvents that are causing the problem, possibly by inhibiting the kidney's retention of potassium, but perhaps the high fluoride content of coffee may be involved somehow as well to some extent.

Vitamin B-3b, niacinamide, has been proposed to alleviate symptoms of rheumatoid arthritis somewhat [http://www.doctoryourself.com/kaufman3. html] This may because it is involved with the synthesis of cortisol. Vitamin B-3 deficiency is likely among people who eat a lot of corn or millet [http:// www.innvista.com/health/nutrition/vitamins/b3.htm].

There is evidence that cetyl myristoleate applied to a certain type of mice reduces the symptoms of arthritis (maybe only osteoarthritis) [Diehl].

It has been proposed that coeliac disease from eating gluten in wheat is more common than thought and may contribute some of Crohn's disease and rheumatoid arthritis [Sinaii] [http://www.guardian.co.uk/medicine/ story/0,11381,793501,00.html]. A genetic inability to digest gluten would not strictly be an allergy, but the damage to the intestines could conceivably affect potassium nutrition and have the affect suggested. It has also been proposed that lectins, or plant proteins which bind certain carbohydrates, contribute to rheumatoid arthritis by enabling antigens [Cordain]. Gluten and concavelin A are lectins.

MEDICINES

Certain herbs have been shown to considerably mute pain and other symptoms of rheumatoid arthritis without side effects. Because they can not be patented there has not been much research on them. I suspect that they are primarily palliative, although interference with potassium excretion has not been explored.

All other medicines that I have heard of are part of hypotheses mentioned above or are pain deadeners.

FUTURE RESEARCH

These hypotheses are not necessarily mutually exclusive and that potassium deficiency is a common thread that runs through many of them is highly probable. Potassium is an element that is essential to every cell in the body. It and sodium are controlled by at least four steroid hormones, several peptide hormones, and some molecular hormones (see chapter 9). It would not be surprising that more than one disease syndrome could arise from a deficiency, especially considering that in addition to that, the twenty five or more essential nutrients are often either deficient or wildly oversupplied in our society as well, in addition to numerous poisons. Considering the last statement it would not be surprising either if fuzzy, inconclusive results were obtained with both nutritional experiments and medication. With such a complicated physiological situation as potassium you must surely see why I will always recommend that nutritional solutions be attempted by eating unprocessed food rather than supplements whenever possible. Food alone may not be sufficient in old people though. Thus imbalances tend to be avoided as well as other deficiencies. In particular it is essential to have adequate magnesium in order to absorb potassium efficiently, and maybe inositol also. Magnesium is part of the chlorophyll in green vegetables. Also a very dangerous imbalance in regard to heart disease can occur if vitamin B-1 is deficient and potassium is supplemented (see chapter 3).

The difficulty in diagnosing arthritis sets doctors up for misdiagnosis. Hemochromatosis (build up of iron in the body) was misdiagnosed as rheumatoid arthritis in the past [Espinosa-Morales], for instance. Most of the recent research has centered around the autoimmune hypothesis or in developing medicines which deaden pain. Unfortunately many of these medicines have had bad effects from the medicines especially on the kidneys or make one susceptible to infection.

These scientific efforts are further thwarted from pursuing nutritional investigations because a certain amount of resistance to new ideas is normal in scientists. Providing the innovations have a means of being tested, there are a number of differences between medicine and pure science that can result in some medical innovations being ignored or rejected without an adequate assessment. Social-organizational factors in medicine appear to favor the acceptance of theoretically glamorous, pharmaceutical, and high technology innovations over simpler and less profitable ones [Forman] even in government research. "There is a principle which is a bar against all information, which is proof against all argument, and which cannot fail to keep man in everlasting ignorance. That principle is condemnation without investigation" (from Herbert Spencer). From the time that cod liver oil was suggested as a treatment for rickets [Schmidt] one hundred and fifty years went by during which cod liver oil actually declined in popularity with the medical profession. It was not until Sir Edward Mellanby established it in 1920 [http://vitamind.ucr.edu/history.html] that it could no longer be denied. Let us hope that we do not have to wait 150 years before potassium is routinely prescribed against rheumatoid arthritis.

CHAPTER 12
CORTISOL

SUMMARY

The primary purpose of cortisol (hydrocortisone) and corticosterone in mammals is to mobilize the body's physiological processes against infection and its adverse effects, cortisol against potassium wasting intestinal disease and corticosterone against scrum disease.. They do this inversely by declining. Cortisol inversely conserves potassium, and loses sodium, conserves water, Cortisol has little affect on glucose and glucagon and no affect on insulin, while corticosterone has a marked inhibition of insulin and stimulation of glucagon. Cortisol inversely stimulates collagen formation and uptake of amino acids by muscle, while inhibiting protein degradation. Both glucocorticoids inversely inhibit gastric secretion. Cortisol inactivates renal glutaminase enzyme generation of ammonium. Net chloride secretion into the intestines is inversely inhibited by cortisol, which negates cholera's affect. Cortisol inversely shuts down most copper containing enzymes to provide copper for immunity. Glucosteroid response modifying factor hormone inhibits most of cortisol's affects when endotoxin containing bacteria attack the body in order to counter that toxin's effects. Some strategies implied by those characteristics are suggested.

This chapter will propose that the primary purpose of cortisol (hydrocortisone) and corticosterone in mammals is to mobilize the body's physiological processes against infection and its adverse effects, cortisol against potassium wasting intestinal disease and corticosterone against serum disease. These steroids control a large number of enzymes, hormones, and processes, most of which could enhance growth of pathogens or make the adverse symptoms worse. The few processes that do not, do not affect immunity either, and are probably opportunistic adaptations of these hormones to peripheral functions. Extinction of juvenile play traits is an example.

Glucocorticoids mobilize immunity by declining their serum concentration. This inverse style is highly desirable, otherwise a pathogen could easily overwhelm the immunity defenses simply by evolving an enzyme which could degrade steroids. Some circumstances controlled inversely enhance an animal's survival from the adverse effects of bacterial poisons or the animal's own defenses. Such a defense would be control of blood pressure. This control, I suspect, is largely to protect infection damaged and copper starved blood vessels from hemorrhage. This inverse concept will be handled in this chapter by using the phrases "inversely inhibits" or inversely stimulates" as cortisol declines.

Cortisol is controlled by the brain pituitary peptide ACTH [Davis]. ACTH is in turn controlled by the hypothalamic peptide, corticotropin releasing factor (CRF) [Plotsky], under nervous control. CRF acts synergisticly with arginine vasopressin, angiotensin II, and epinephrine [Plotsky]. Therefore ACTH and CRF cannot be overwhelmed by bacterial degradation either. ACTH probably controls cortisol by controlling movement of calcium into the cortisol secreting target cells [Davis].

Cortisol prevents proliferation of T-cells by rendering the interleukin-2 producer T-cells unresponsive to interleukin-1 (IL-1), and unable to produce the T-cell growth factor [Palacios]. That cortisol often increases during infection does not make this hypothesis invalid because when activated macrophages start to secrete interleukin-1, which synergistically with corticotrophin releasing factor (CRF) increase ACTH [Besedovsky 1986] [Besedovsky 1984], T-cells also secrete glucosteroid response modifying factor (GRMF) as well as interleukin-1, both of which increase the amount of cortisol required to inhibit almost all the immune cells [Fairchild] (I have seen no information in the literature that indicates whether glucosteroid response modifying factor is the same as transcortin, also called cortisol binding globulin (CBG), or not. See an article by Torpy for what the CBG molecule is thought to look like and some of its action [Torpy]. It is the same as glucocorticoids antagonizing factor or GAF). Thus immune cells take over their own regulation, but at a higher set point. Even so, the rise of cortisol in diarrheic calves is minimal over healthy calves and drops below with time [Dvorak]. The cells do not lose all of the fight or flight override because of interleukin-1's synergism with CRF (corticotrpin releasing factor). Cortisol even has a negative feedback affect on interleukin-1 [Besedovsky 1986] which must be especially useful against those diseases that gain an advantage by forcing the hypothalamus to secrete corticotrophin releasing factor, such as the endotoxin bacteria to be discussed later.

The suppressor cells are not affected by glucosteroid response modifying factor [Fairchild], so that the effective set point for the immune cells may be even higher than the set point for physiological processes. It may be that the glucosteroid response modifying factor has a different spectrum of effects for each of the physiological processes in order to fine tune the immune response in order to optimize the attack against different organisms. Glucocorticosteroid response modifying factor (called GAF in this reference) primarily affects the liver rather than the kidneys for some physiological processes [Stith],

Natural killer cells are not affected by cortisol [Onsrud]. This would be logical for a hormone that is used to fight intestinal disease, not scrum disease. Also cortisol (as dexamethasone, a close man made similar molecule) also has additive affects on inhibition of TH1 cytokine (antiviral) production when combined with vitamin D. However, vitamin D has no affect on cortisol's affect on TH2 cytokines (antibacterial) [Jirapongsananuruk]. This further hints that cortisol is involved with bacterial disease, because the body has evolved no affect by a vitamin D deficiency on anti bacterial cytokines.

It seems to me that resources diverted to immunity or denied to non-viral pathogens usually diminish an animal's performance when fighting or fleeing. Therefore, the cortisol system can be overridden by perceived danger. This is no doubt made desirable because it takes several hours or more for pathogens to rise to dangerous levels, but only a few seconds for a predator to kill an animal. Anxiety is also factored in because, I suggest, cortisol operates by changing the nucleus commands to send RNA out for production of enzymes, etc. in almost every case and the various diffusion steps take an hour or more to complete. Therefore, an anticipation of danger would be very desirable. This is no doubt a considerable part of the mechanism behind the placebo role in experiments.

The desirability of inhibiting activity during infection is no doubt the reason why cortisol is responsible for creating euphoria [Newsholme, p736]], as does aldosterone [Mach], and presumably the reverse upon declining. The desirability of not disturbing tissues weakened by infection or of not cutting off their blood supply could explain the inverse stimulation of pain widely observed for cortisol. These neural mechanisms as geared to stress have been emphasized in concepts concerning glucocorticoids as pioneered by Selye up to now. Nevertheless, when a process must move in the same direction for both immunity and fight or flight, a different hormone system controls it for stress. An example is release of ceruloplasmin by the liver, which is controlled for purposes of stress by epinephrine and by an unknown hormone for immunity to be discussed later.

The most dangerous digestive diseases produce a protein poison which stimulates cyclic adenosine monophosphate (c-AMP) hormone in such a way that the intestines cannot remove water from their contents [Mekalanos] and thus cause diarrhea. Since potassium in food and the 2.5 grams or so secreted with digestive fluids can only move into the blood stream passively [Kernon], this causes a large loss of potassium. Judging by the reduction of the death rate in babies with virulent diarrhea from 34% to 6% by potassium supplements [Govan] in spite of the danger of hyperkalemia (high serum potassium) during dehydration, the loss of potassium implied is the most serious consequence of diarrhea. When this poison first evolved, it must have been catastrophic to terrestrial vertebrates. Even today, after what was probably a major evolutionary transformation of cortisol during many tens of millions of years, the diarrheas are among the most important causes of mortality in the tropics, especially cholera [Colwell], and diarrhea was the third leading cause of death 100 or so years ago in the USA, ahead of heart disease. Even currently a virus called rotovirus kills 600,000 children each year, most of the deaths in India, sub Sahara Africa, and western Africa [Glass]. It must have been imperative to evolve mechanisms to surmount those pathogens. In most mammals, a wide range of processes are stimulated by cortisol, each of which would make an animal less able to resist potassium and water wasting intestinal disease. Rodents have very little or no cortisol, which may have been made possible by a marked inhibition of the affect of cholera toxin on rodents' intestinal contents [Donowitz]. Also, c-AMP increases water absorption in their ascending colon, opposite to the effect in their descending colon [Hornyck]. This makes rodents dubious for experiments on the hypothalamic-adrenal axis and perhaps for any experiments. These attributes are possibly one reason why rodents have more vertebrate species than any order [Meng] and why they are so well adapted to desert life.

POTASSIUM

The greatest urgency during diarrhea is to prevent loss of potassium, because there is no storage of potassium in any cell. In cells, 88% of the potassium is in free solution [Kernan]. Indeed, one of cortisol's functions conserves potassium. It has been suggested that cortisol tends to move potassium inversely into the cells (cortisone used instead of cortisol) [Knight]. Sodium load augments the intense potassium excretion by cortisol, and corticosterone is comparable to cortisol in this case [Muller]. Because this is the case, potassium is inversely conserved by lower secretion of cortisol (dexamethasone used) [Bia]. This is no doubt the reason why a potassium deficiency has evolved to cause cortisol to decline [Mikosha] and why a potassium deficiency causes a decrease in conversion of 11deoxycortisol to cortisol [Bauman]. Without this the body would have no way of knowing that there was an infection in the intestines other than perhaps dehydration. In order for potassium to move into the cell, cortisol inversely moves out an equal number of sodium ions [Knight]. It can be seen that this should make pH regulation much easier, unlike the normal potassium deficiency situation in which about 2 sodium ions move in for each 3 potassium ions that move out [Weber 1983, p445], which is closer to the DOC effect [Knight]. This is probably the main reason why the cell becomes more acid during a deficiency caused by low potassium intake [Gardner]. Nevertheless, cortisol consistently causes alkalosis of the serum (inversely acidosis) while in a potassium deficiency pH (alkalinity) does not change. I suspect that this may be for the purpose of bringing serum pH to a value most optimum for some of the immune enzymes.

Potassium is also inversely inhibited from loss in the kidneys somewhat by cortisol (using 9 alpha fluorohydrocortisone) [Barger]. However potassium is primarily blocked from loss in the kidneys by a drastic decline of aldosterone during dehydration [Schneider] [Dollman]. Aldosterone acts on the last part of the kidney tubules and the lower colon. In the colon, aldosterone reverses the normal inward flow of potassium, or at least stops its reabsorption [Adler] and so inversely conserves potassium there. Aldosterone is directly controlled by potassium and inversely by osmotic pressure [Schneider] while angiotensin II is required. Thus as osmotic pressure rises during dehydration, aldosterone undergoes a drastic decline. Aldosterone also backs up cortisol by possibly inversely moving potassium into muscle cells somewhat [Adler].

To be useful in combating a potassium wasting disease, it would be necessary for cortisol to decline at such a time. A high potassium media, which stimulates aldosterone secretion in vitro, also stimulates cortisol secretion from the fasciculata zone of dog adrenals [Mikosha]. and potassium loading increases ACTH and cortisol in people [101]. Therefore, low potassium should decrease cortisol secretion by the adrenals in dogs and people. At the same time, potassium has no affect on corticosterone secreted by the adrenal fasciculate [Mendelsohn]. Since the fasciculata accounts for 5/8 of the corticosterone secreted, the net effect is very little decline in corticosterone secretion. This is evidence that the body does not rely on corticosterone against diarrhea. Potassium chloride supplements do not affect cortisol or corticosterone plasma concentrations in humans in vivo when the cell content is adequate [Scholer]. I know of no experiment which would establish the effect of potassium, cholera toxin or detection of intestinal pathogen microbes on ACTH. ACTH has its greatest affect on cortisol and 18hydroxy 11 deoxycorticosterone [18OH DOC]. That last affect on hormones may be to increase the acidity of the serum or, perhaps more likely, to permit potassium loss as dehydration makes it necessary by eliminating the interference of hydrogen ion with potassium excretion.

SODIUM

Cortisol is used to stimulate sodium inward for fresh water fish and outward for salt-water fish [Sandle]. The necessity of conserving potassium while still unloading electrolytes to maintain osmotic pressure, may explain cortisol's inverse sodium losing power in the small intestine in mammals [Sandle]. By using the intestine to excrete sodium, less water is needed for kidney processes, which is crucial during diarrhea. Sodium depletion does not affect cortisol [Mason], so cortisol is not used to regulate serum sodium. It is known that the sodium retaining hormone, 18-hydroxy 11-deoxycorticosterone [18OH DOC] acting on the kidneys is strongly dependent on ACTH. When ACTH sinks to zero, 18OH DOC also does [Tan]. Therefore, it also is inversely involved in unloading sodium in what little water is excreted from the kidneys. The need for sodium chloride by diarrhea bacteria in order to grow rapidly [Doyle] may be the main reason why cholera enterotoxin is so successful for this bacterium and of course increased water undoubtedly assists it also. 18OH DOC is probably the hormone which stimulates hydrogen ion excretion [Weber 1983], so loss of this excretion would assist acidifying the serum as mentioned above as well.

If my contention that 16-alpha 18-dihydroxy 11-deoxycorticosterone (DOH-DOC) [Weber 1983] is relied on to excrete excess sodium and to conserve potassium is valid, it should follow that ACTH and/or cortisol either have no affect on DOH-DOC or, possibly more usefully, to inversely stimulate it. It should also be desirable for DOH-DOC to exert its affect in the intestines because in nature it is almost always during diarrhea that the body experiences a potassium deficiency and sodium glut. I have no direct evidence for either phenomenon. However, it is known that DOH-DOC has very little affect on the kidneys [Weber 1983, p446]. The malaise, headache, loss of appetite, insomnia, and muscle cramps created by DOC injections [Relman] may be due to the loss of potassium and retention of sodium, resulting from increased DOC, causing DOH-DOC to rise, since none of these symptoms appear from a high sodium and potassium diet which stimulates DOC [Weber 1983]. Some of those attributes would be useful during diarrhea, but I have no evidence for DOH-DOC's role. 11-deoxycorticosterone [DOC] is the only steroid left of the four I proposed for electrolyte regulation [Weber 1983]. Sodium retention must never completely disappear. This may be why, as possibly the only renal sodium retainer left, DOC has acquired its auxiliary powers with respect to amino acids and copper to be discussed later and why a fall in leucocyte potassium of over 10% is observed from DOC [Wilson] and a decline in muscle potassium [Tobian], thus joining cortisol in inversely conserving potassium. It also probably explains why it is mediated partly by ACTH since ACTH must surely largely be an immune hormone with stress as an adjunct [Weber 1983, p445].

WATER

Cortisol also acts as a water diuretic hormone. Half the intestinal diuresis is so controlled [Sandle]. Kidney diuresis is also controlled by cortisol in dogs [Boylin]. The decline in water excretion upon decline of cortisol [dexamethasone] in dogs is probably due to inverse stimulation of antidiuretic hormone (ADH or arginine vasopressin) the inverse stimulation of which is not overridden by water loading. Humans also use this mechanism [Dingman] and other different animal mechanisms operate in the same direction.

Because loss of water is the circumstance which produces the worst adverse effects of diarrhea, it would seem to be logical to use dehydration as a signal to decrease cortisol. Cortisol has been found to vary directly with water intake [Gutenbrunner]. ACTH hormone production is inhibited by water deprivation at the pituitary level. Base secretion of ACTH is not affected, but high plasma ACTH resulting from immobilization stress is almost cut in half. Base corticosterone is increased in plasma from dehydration, but the much higher corticosterone from immobilization stress is not affected by water status [Aguilera]. The above is additional evidence that corticosterone is used by the body to fight serum disease and cortisol is used to fight intestinal disease.

GLUCOSE

Reinforcing the concept that cortisol is relied on more for intestinal disease control and corticosterone for serum disease is the circumstance that corticosterone at physiological levels shows a marked inhibition of insulin and enhancement of glucagon in vitro [Barseghian & Devine]. Cortisol shows a small inhibition of glucagon which reverses in a short time and has no affect on insulin [Barseghian, Rashmid, & Epps]. Insulin is used to help prevent hyperkalemia [high serum potassium] by the body. As glucose moves into the cell, it takes potassium with it. This mechanism is only used at low potassium intakes. At an intake of 8 grams per day, insulin stays normal [Knochel]. This is logical since there is no need to conserve potassium at high intakes and aldosterone is relied on to lower serum potassium. Cortisone greatly inhibits insulin secretion [Barseghian, Rashmid, & Epps]. The cortisone-cortisol equilibrium may explain why in vivo experiments contradict the above [Curry]. It is possible that this equilibrium may permit the body to change cortisol glucose responses for particular kinds of situations.

The inversed stimulation of insulin by corticosterone would lower serum glucose and thus deny glucose to pathogens. Such an aptitude in cortisol would be of little value if my thesis is correct, and could even endanger an animal from hypokalemia [low serum potassium] during diarrhea. A sudden withdrawal of glucose by insulin in a potassium deficiency can lower serum potassium enough to be lethal. However, apparently there is an advantage in locking up the potassium that does enter the cell in a more orderly manner with glycogen, because DOC inversely stimulates glycogen formation [Bartlett]. Cortisol does inversely cause serum glucose to fall, but this is probably an indirect effect caused by inverse inhibition of amino acid degradation.

The intestinal brush border disaccharide enzymes are inversely inhibited by cortisone [Yeh]. If it is cortisol that is actually involved, this could be a mechanism to deny energy to bacteria incapable of using sucrose. However, present day cholera can ferment sucrose [Finkelstein, p557] so it would have to be an attribute developed against diarrheas which evolved before cholera evolved. It is also possible that it helps prevent the hypokalemia above or make copper more available if those enzymes are copper catalyzed. The fact that sucrose and fructose make a copper deficiency much worse suggests that they are [Reiser].

AMINO ACIDS

Glucocorticoids have the attribute of inversely lowering amino acids in the serum [Manchester, p273]. They do this by inversely stimulating collagen formation, increasing amino acid uptake by muscle, and stimulating protein synthesis [Manchester, p273]. Cortisol also inversely inhibits protein degradation. Such an attribute would help deny amino acids to bacteria. An additional advantage is that collagen can be very useful in repair of infected tissue. An indication of this last is that loss of collagen from skin by cortisol is ten times greater than from all other tissue in the rat (collagen normally has a half life of one year) [Houck]. Thus the skin can be a reasonably safe source of energy during stress and be rapidly repaired during damage preliminary to or caused by infection. Lowering serum amino acid or even tissue damage repair during intestinal disease should be not nearly so advantageous. An indication that it is not is that DOC acts in the opposite direction for collagen [mice] [Popsilova] and thus tends to cancel cortisol's effect if the same thing happens in other animals.

It can be seen that denying amino acids to bacteria above could be very advantageous in a serum infection. However, the inverse generalized stimulation of protein synthesis [Manchester, p273] (I'm not certain how generalized it is) could have additional survival rationale against digestive disease. 40% of the protein synthesis is in the intestines of the rat, much of it for synthesis of IgA [Newby]. IgA acts as an inert, non lethal coating on bacteria to prevent adhesion to intestinal walls [Newby] and is the predominant immunoglobulin in the human intestine [Finkelstein, p597]. Its production depends on the vitamin A metabolite, retinoic acid [Mora]. Mora, et al, discuss how specialized B cells from lymphoid tissue associated with the intestines migrate to the intestines' wall where interleukin 5 and 6 peptide hormones permit retinoic acid to stimulate secretion of IgA [Mora, p1160]. This is no doubt the reason why vitamin A supplements decrease mortality from diarrhea by 34% in malnourished children [Mora]. Cortisol (as opticortinol) probably inversely stimulates IgA precursor cells in the intestines of calves [Husband]. Cortisol also inversely stimulates IgA in serum, as it does IgM, but not IgE [Posey], although serum IgA does not depend on vitamin A. I cannot account for the affects on IgM and IgE.

Cortisol has an opposite affect on liver than it has on muscle, but I cannot tie this for sure into the immune concept now. I suspect that it may be to provide a small amount of maintenance amino acids when the muscles are withdrawing them from the blood and possibly also to provide liver amino acids for IgA. That same inability of mine is true of its inverse activation of luteinizing hormone.

HYDROGEN ION OR ACIDITY

Sodium and potassium make strong bases, and chloride strong acid so that any unilateral movement by any of them has considerable implications in hydrogen ion control (acid and alkaline). Cortisol inversely inhibits gastric acid secretion [Soffer]. Since hydrogen ion interferes with potassium excretion at the kidneys [Welt, p215], this could be having a potassium conserving effect, especially since gastric secretion carries 0.6 grams of potassium per day into the stomach as well. Corticosterone has a much greater affect on gastric acid secretion than cortisol [Soffer]. I cannot explain why it should have any affect at all unless there is some advantage to keeping the serum at a lower pH during infection for enzyme enhancement, a possibility already mentioned. Some leucocyte enzymes have a pH optimum lower than serum. If so, 18hydroxy-11deoxycorticosterone, which reduces bicarbonate and stimulates hydrogen ion excretion at the kidneys [Damasco], operates in the same direction, since it also declines with ACTH half again more than cortisol [Delkers]. Cortisol's only direct affect on the hydrogen ion excretion of the kidneys is to inversely inhibit excretion of ammonium ion by inactivation of renal glutaminase enzyme [Kokshchuk]. Glutaminase splits ammonia off of the amino acid glutamic acid, and this provides ammonium ion to take the place of potassium for excretion. However, cortisol's presence is necessary for the other hydrogen ion excretion regulator to operate [Kokshchuk]. There would have to be some restraint on hydrogen ion loss because when potassium is deficient, the kidneys fail to absorb chloride and the serum tends toward alkalosis [Luks]. Perhaps cortisol's inverse inhibition of gastric secretion being lower than corticosterone's is a compromise made necessary by the advantage in keeping the stomach reasonably acid, below a pH of 6, in order to help prevent reinfection by cholera bacteria, since cholera bacteria are sensitive to acid below a pH of 6.0 [Finkelstein, p556]. The acidosis of serum that attends cholera [Finkelstein. P601] may become too high, so this lower inhibition may also be a compromise to help solve such a situation. The net affect of glucocorticoids is to inversely acidify the serum.

CHLORIDE

Chloride is intimately involved with potassium loss because when the cell loses potassium to take the place of serum losses and sodium migrates in, chloride must also be excreted as the only ion which has a chance of maintaining serum pH. In a potassium deficiency chloride is lost [Luks]. This is a serious circumstance in terrestrial nature because chloride is not bound very well by soils. It is a seriously limiting element inland where vegetation is devoid of it as a rule. Some indication of its importance is that it is the only essential nutrient we can detect and be attracted to other than water [the salty taste].

Net chloride secretion in the intestines is inversely decreased by cortisol in vitro (as methylprednisolone) [Tai]. Cholera toxin forces chloride secretion to reverse from flow inward, to larger flow outward [Field]. Thus cortisol tends to inversely neutralize cholera's effect. There is no net movement of chloride by cholera toxin in vivo [Charnes]. It is possible that this attribute is related to keeping the serum pH low as mentioned above, that is to say, acidic. It is possible that movement of sodium and/or chloride into the intestines is the chief advantage that diarrhea bacteria attempt to gain from their water losing toxin.

COPPER

The immune system is very sensitive to copper availability. Spleen of copper deficient animals shows little growth during infections [Weber 1984, p334]. Even a mild deficiency causes spleen derived immune cells to be significantly less competent as stimulators in general and also to be stimulated by endotoxin, pokeweed, or concanavalin A [Lukaseqvcz]. Resistance to infection is reduced somewhat by a deficiency [Weber 1984, p334]. A reduction in neutrophils is the first symptom of a deficiency in children [Weber 1984, p336].

It is therefore probable that increasing copper for immune purposes is the reason why many copper enzymes are inversely inhibited to an extent which is often 50% of their total potential by cortisol [Weber 1984, p337]. This includes lysyl oxidase, an enzyme which is used to cross link collagen and elastin [Weber 1084, p334]. DOC acts in the same direction as cortisol for lysyl oxidase [Weber 1084, p337]. Particularly valuable for immunity is the inverse shutdown of superoxide dismutase by cortisol [Flohe], because this copper enzyme is almost certainly used by the body to inversely permit superoxide to poison bacteria. Superoxide is lethal to cholera [Ghosh]. Indication that superoxide dismutase is involved in immunity is that phagocytic activity is reduced by free radical scavengers [Smith].

The safest way to transport copper to the immune system would be by the transport protein, ceruloplasmin [Weber 1985, p335]. This avoids copper toxicity when it is necessary for copper availability to the cells from the liver be increased, because ceruloplasmin copper is not in equilibrium with the serum [Weber 1984, p335]. The concept that ceruloplasmin is used by the immune cells as a source of copper is supported by the fact that ceruloplasmin quadruples in replete chickens during infection [Starch] and several antigens raise plasma ceruloplasmin in mammals [Starch] by an unknown hormone, which has been tentatively proposed to be leucocyte endogenous mediator, at low ACTH levels [Evans p557]. Cortisol is not used to inversely stimulate ceruloplasmin. I suspect the reason why cortisol is not used is that stress requires extra copper, also, and at high ACTH levels epinephrine is used for this purpose [Evans p556]. Transporting copper as the ion is not so important for denying copper to pathogens during digestive disease, which is probably why DOC inversely loses copper from the liver and inhibits liver uptake somewhat thus providing the immune cells with free copper to supplement the ceruloplasmin source [Gregordiadis]. Some might argue that it is not likely that the immune cells depend on ceruloplasmin since people with Wilson's disease, in whom ceruloplasmin cannot be synthesized, are not prone to infection. However, such people cannot transport copper to the bile excretory proteins either, so their cells are already loaded and even overloaded with copper.

Cortisol causes an inverse four or five fold decrease of metallothionein [Piletz], a copper storage protein. This may be to furnish more copper for ceruloplasmin synthesis. Cortisol has an opposite affect on alpha aminoisobuteric acid than on the other amino acids [Chambers]. If alpha aminoisobuteric acid is used to transport copper through the intestine's cell wall and thus away from diarrhea bacteria, this anomaly would possibly be explained.

MISCELLANEOUS

A large number of other molecules and processes are affected by glucocorticoids which I cannot tie into the immune system definitively at this time. A cursory examination has revealed none to me that are at variance with this thesis. They include smell sensitivity, fear, taste of chloride, pain, appetite, fever, immune cell activity, prostaglandins through arachidonic acid availability, fibronectins, capillary permeability, calcium absorption, intestinal permeability, phosphate, depression, oxidation of chloride, free oxygen formation, blood platelet activating factor, T-cell growth factor sensitivity, and lysosome membrane. Some of these are thought to be controlled by a second message protein, lipocortin, via its affect on phospholipases [Hirahata].

ENDOTOXIN

Many gram negative bacteria have evolved a very potent way of subverting the cortisol control of immunity. They have a lipopolysacharride called endotoxin on their cell wall. Some endotoxin erodes off the wall and more is released into the blood stream when polymorpholeucocytes eject debris from bacteria which they have engulfed [Devoe]. The lipid A part of the endotoxin molecule stimulates the hypothalamus to secrete large amounts of corticotrophin releasing factor. An amount of endotoxin which causes no other symptoms than a mild fever causes a six fold rise in ACTH, undoubtedly from corticotrophin releasing factor stimulation [Melby]. Activity appears one hour after endotoxin enters the blood, is at a maximum by 2 hours, and is almost undetectable by 3-4 hours [Moore, Goodrun, etc.]. Tumor necrosing factor (TNF) appears at the same time, the same fraction, and the same heat sensitivity [Moore, Goodrun, etc.] [extended discussion in Moore, ; Shackleford, & Berry]. When this way of bypassing ACTH immunity control first arose, it must have been catastrophic for vertebrate life.

A way of detecting endotoxin has apparently evolved and, also, a way of using it to activate a number of responses, some of which are reminiscent of glucocorticoids' inverse affects. Some responses are fever, creation of interferon by spleen cells as well as division of spleen cells, synthesis of IL-6, activation of complement by three mechanisms, creation of hypotension (low blood pressure), stimulation of adherence and oxidative processes of neutrophiles, activation of a burst of activity in macrophages in extremely small amounts, proliferation and maturation of B-cells, suppression of cholera toxin, low serum glucose, metabolic acidosis, and numerous other functions [Beutler &

Cerami A]. Mice which lack these capabilities are susceptible to gram negative disease [Beutler & Cerami A]. Most of these responses are mediated by the peptide hormone, tumor necrosing factor (TNF, cacectin, cachexin) secreted by macrophages and they last only the first couple of hours [Beutler & Cerami C]. That the detection and cathectin system evolved after the endotoxin assault on ACTH evolved is indicated by the much different appearance of the response curve for endotoxin as opposed to TNF [Michle]. If both TNF and gamma interferon are removed by antibodies, bacteria proliferate very rapidly to the host's death. Lipid A fraction of endotoxin enhances local IgA response to mucosally applied antigen (cholera toxin), at least when lipid A and antigen are associated on a liposome carrier [Pierce]. GRMFs' (glucocorticosteroid response modifying factors, which are probably glycoproteins) secretions are stimulated by endotoxin [Mishel]. Antidiuretic hormone quickly rises twenty fold in only 15 minutes [Oyama]. Endotoxin must therefore be acting directly on the source of this hormone through TNF, in my view by a secondary evolutionary response of the hosts. Thus, the body forces endotoxin to mount a preliminary quick response even before the antigens can activate a response, and then quickly turns it off again assisted by a TNF half life of only six minutes [Hall].

The release of endotoxin by phagocytosis mentioned above is probably the reason why glucocorticoids inhibit digestion but not uptake of bacteria by macrophages [Mannel]. This mechanism probably gives the body time to mount its TNF, glucocorticoid response modifying factor, antibody to endotoxin, and other defenses before the endotoxin containing cell walls are released into the serum.

It would be advantageous if ACTH production could be cut off when under attack. Possibly two proteins detoxify endotoxin [Johnson]. Apparently, a mechanism has evolved to cause endotoxin to lose its ability to force ACTH secretion in a few hours [Jones]. This loss may be difficult to control because lymphocytes have developed the ability to secrete a protein, interleukin 1 (IL-1), which has a function of stimulating cortisol secretion [Besedovsky 1984, book], which it does indirectly by stimulating corticotropin releasing factor (CRF) [Uehara], as does IL-6 (the mode of IL-6 action is unknown to me). In other words, the immune system takes over its own regulation. Such a system would be necessary if the ACTH decline were severe because even the immune system cells require maintenance amounts of glucocorticoids. Those glucocorticoid hormones cause the immune cells to rise to a peak of activity at low concentrations and then decline again at increasing concentrations [Finlay]. The IL-1 system has an excellent negative feedback [Besedovsky 1986]. IL-1 still retains at least part of the fight or flight override, because it is synergistic with CRF in its long term effects. TNF also stimulates ACTH production somewhat by a direct affect on the pituitary [Milenkovic], possibly an advantage the first few hours, especially if the shutdown of ACTH is rapid.

GLUCOSTEROID RESPONSE MODIFYING FACTOR

It would seem desirable if the excess cortisol could be destroyed and, indeed, the half life of cortisol becomes markedly reduced [Besedovsky 1986]. What really makes the IL-1 system practical, however, is the development of a glycoprotein produced by T-cells called glucocorticoid response modifying factor (GRMF, also GAF), which along with IL-1 has the power to inhibit the response of immune cells to cortisol [Fairchild] In other words, the set point of cortisol is raised. Thus, the now multiple sources of ACTH stimulation can be accommodated.

The GRMF system has taken on an advantage not enjoyed by the previous cortisol only control. Since GRMF does not inhibit cortisol's affect on the immune suppressor cells [Fairchild], as previously mentioned, the other immune cells must be stepped up to an even greater frenzy. I suspect a primary pressure forcing the evolution of this system was the advent of endotoxin. The pressure must have been intense because some very virulent diseases are endotoxin involved. They include cholera, typhoid, pneumonia, salmonella, campylobacter, and meningitis. Non-gram negative malaria may also synthesize endotoxin [Clark] perhaps, but if so, probably by some ancient recombinant gene event. Evidence has not been obtained yet that GRMFs affect most of the physiological processes affected by cortisol other than immune cell activity. However GRMF does block phosphoenolpyruvate and fails to block Dibutyryl cyclic AMP induced enzyme synthesis and tyrosine aminotransferase [Goodrun]. I am not familiar enough with these systems to be able to comment on the significance of these phenomena to the immune system.

CONCLUSIONS

If glucocorticoids are truly immunocorticoids as suggested, it should be possible to use existing information to devise strategies for dealing with infection. It would seem likely that keeping the patient free of stressful thoughts and actions [http://stress.about.com/od/stresshealth/a/cortisol.htm], warm [Portanova], on a low food intake (except maybe for virus), and on a high copper intake (prior to infection) would be advantageous. One way to decrease stress seems to be by way of massage [Field]. It is possible that refraining from coffee, tea, soft drinks or cocoa would prove slightly advantageous also because of an affect on cortisol by caffeine [De Pasquale].

If the patient cannot be guarded from stress, then vitamin C (ascorbic acid) supplements would probably be useful, for they are said to have the effect of blocking a rise in corticosterone resulting from stress [Civen]. There is a discussion of diseases for which vitamin C would be advantageous [http://www.orthomed.com/], for some, very advantageous. The advantage may disappear at other times because corticosterone is said to rise some, normally [Civen]. Making sure the patient has ample water during serum disease is probably advantageous because of the affect water status has on corticosterone as mentioned under "Water". Fasting at the noon meal may prove to be a good strategy since cortisol shows a surge then if one eats, but not at the evening meal [Quigley].

Also, 250 watt infrared heat lamps creating an artificial very high fever [Hanson] [Kluger] [Weber 2007], directly on the infected part (except for fungae [personal observation]), probably are very effective. The immune system is stimulated by a rise in temperature. This could be a response arising by interleuken-1 [Hanson]. This has been demonstrated for interleukin-1 and interleukin-2 in post operative hypothermia [Beilin]. Heat also stimulates tumor necrosis factor (TNF) [Zellner]. It could be the reason why the ability to create a fever arose [Kluger]. Doubling time of pneumococcal meningitis in rabbits is increased at fever temperature, and that bacteria did not grow at all at 41 degrees centigrade in either soy broth or cerebral fluid [Small]. So it seems that the efficacy of body temperature effectiveness is dependent on more than enhancement of the immune system. It is conceivable in view of their results that rather than the fever evolving in order to enhance an innate characteristic of the immune system, the fever evolved to take advantage of an innate ineffectiveness of most bacteria at high temperatures and the immune system evolved to be most effective during a fever. It is important to create an artificial fever as soon as possible, because it is most effective early on [Bell].

The efficacies of these strategies should be established as soon as possible with controlled experiments on primates and made known to the public early on. Such experiments would prove to be very cost effective indeed compared to hospitalization. To rely on hunches based on knowledge of similar chemistry, old wives' tales, and alterations of symptoms by chemicals, such as even the medical profession does currently, is sad and inane. Few will alter their life styles unless they are convinced that the matter is established. It is highly desirable that the theory behind any parameter be understood because even small variations in the patient's environment can sometimes make an otherwise desirable strategy backfire. Nutrition intake and ingestion of poisons and medicines vary wildly in our society, so that treatments based solely on empirical studies such as is the usual case at present in the medical profession can be more than mildly disadvantageous in particular instances.

It simply is not possible to take anything for granted in the absence of an experiment. I strongly suspect that the current attitude of the medical profession that potassium can never be deficient, or that rheumatoid arthritis can not possibly be a chronic potassium deficiency even though no experiment has ever been reported (until Rastmanesh's recent experiment [Rastmanesh]), will prove to be tragically wrong, for instance.

In addition, there seems to me to be implied possibilities for clinical intervention against virulent diseases. A recombinant produced antibody against ACTH or CRF could conceivably have considerable value early in diseases which force their secretion. Perhaps even more valuable and safer would be an antibody against endotoxin. Infection is like a waste paper basket fire. It should be snuffed early before it becomes a raging inferno. Recombinant glucosteroid response modifying factor might also prove valuable early in almost any disease. Where glucosteroid response modifying factor might prove invaluable at all stages could be in those diseases which compromise the T-cells, such as AIDS, and thus hopefully solve the possible relative excess of glucocorticoids in AIDS [Da Prate]. Of course, the frequency of injections for peptides must take into account the half life of the peptide in order to be effective. Massive daily doses would be ineffective, and possibly dangerous in most cases. Ceruloplasmin injections would probably be in order for people known to be in a copper deficiency during serum diseases.

It seems conceivable that if a strain of cholera bacteria could be developed which could not synthesize c-AMP toxin or any other toxin, encapsulated in enteric tablets in order to bypass the stomach acids, and swallowed in large amounts, it could act as a preventative to cholera during an epidemic by furnishing overwhelming competition to virulent cholera in the intestines. It might even be effective after an infection.

In any case, it seems to me to be very foolish to administer cortisol to any class of people whose immune system is known to be weak, such as rheumatoid arthritics. If it is desired to raise cortisol's affect in the body, why not use something safe like potassium supplements, or better and safer yet, leafy, unboiled vegetables? At the same time, it would solve the problem of the other affects of low whole body potassium content which consistently afflicts a large number of people. Rheumatoid arthritics have normal cortisol [http://rheumatology.oupjournals.org/cgi/reprint/38/4/298] so the lower number of glucocorticosteroid receptors [Schlaghecke], or possibly an abnormal glucosteroid response modifying factor secretion, must be involved, perhaps triggered by the potassium deficiency itself or some poison. Attempting to solve the problem by injecting cortisol for more than a short time strikes me as being dangerous. As mentioned in chapter 11 one author summed it up thus "It is amazing how effective cortisol is in getting a seemingly hopeless patient on his feet again. Sometimes it is so effective that he can walk all the way to the autopsy table". Cortisol is not a medicine, it is a hormone, a hormone the effects of which ramify through multiple functions in most of the cell groups in the body. An indication of how fundamental it is, is that the liver's RNA synthesis in adrenalectomized rats is simulated 2-3 fold by cortisol [Kinney].

The immune system is extremely important to us, so current exploration of immunity should continue on by all known means. However, as you explore, please differentiate between cortisol and corticosterone, use the natural versions, use physiological quantities for at least part of the experiment, use animals other than rodents, and translate jargon. As to this last, immunity is important and extremely complicated. Few scientists are expert in all phases of it and all vocabulary. In particular, I suggest you use only well known acronyms.

Under no circumstances should recombinant experiments be performed which give to any microbe the ability to synthesize cortisol, ACTH, CRF, or any hormone molecule which declines in concentration or effecta during infection. No recombinant experiment of any kind should be performed on any microbe which synthesizes endotoxin, such as Escheriischia coli. There are thousands of other species.

Of course there is little point to performing endless research if we have no intention of using the information anyway, as the criminally incompetent food processors are currently failing to so utilize when they add poisons to food or remove essential nutrients..

CHAPTER 13
POTASSIUM IN FOOD TABLE,
ALPHABETICAL ORDER

Potassium is expressed as milligrams per Calorie, which is the most useful form.

Almonds, 1.3—apples, 1.9—apple butter, 1.4—apple juice, 2.1— apricots, raw, 5.5— apricots, canned, no sugar 6.5—apricots, frozen, sweetened 2.3—apricots necter, 2.7— asparagus, raw, 10.1— asparagus, boiled, 9.1— aspargras, canned, solids and liquids, 9.2—asparagras, frozen, 10.4—avocados, 3.6— baby food cereal, high protein, 3.0— custard pudding, 0.9— fruit pudding, 0.8—apple sauce, Bacon, fried, 0.4—Bacon, Canadian, fried, 1.8—Bamboo shoots, 19.8— bananas, 4.4—Barley, 0.5—Bass, sea, 2.8—BEAN SEEDS (white, raw, 3.5—red,raw, 2.9—lima raw, 5.3—lima, boiled 3.8—lima, canned, drained 2.3—lima, canned & liquid 3.1—lima, frozen 4.8—lima, frozen, baby 3.6)—Beans, mung, sprouted 6.4—Beans, sprouted, mung, boiled 5.6—beans green snap (raw 7.6— boiled, short time, minimum water 6.0—boiled, long time much water 6.0—canned, with liquid 5.3—canned, solids only 4.0—canned, liquid 9.5—canned, low sodium with liquid 5.9—frozen 6.4)—beef broiled or roast (chuck, 18% fat 1.1—hamburger, lean 2.6—hamburger, regular 1.6—corned, medium fat 0.4—chipped, cooked, creamed 1.0)—Beer 0.6—Beets, raw 7.8—Beets, cooked 6.5—Beets, canned, & liquid 4.9—Beet greens 23.7—Blackberries 2.9—Blueberries, raw 1.3—Blueberries, canned 0.8—Blueberries, canned with syrup 0.4—Blueberries, frozen 1.5—Blueberries, frozen with syrup 0.6—Bouillion cubes 0.8 {sodium=200.0}—Brains, all kinds 1.6—Bran, with sugar & malt 4.4—Bran flakes 3.0—Brazilnuts 1.1—breads (cracked wheat 0.5—pumpernickel 1.8—rye 0.6—white, 6% dry milk 0.4)—Broccoli, raw 12.0—Broccoli, frozen 8.7—Broccoli, frozen, boiled 8.5—Brussels sprouts, raw 8.7—Brussels sprouts, frozen 9.1—Brussels sprouts, frozen, boiled 8.9—Buckwheat, whole 1.8—Butter 0.0—Buttermilk 3.9—Cabbage, raw 9.0—Cabbage, shredded, boiled, little water 8.1—Cabbage, wedges, boiled 8.4—Cake, angelfood 0.3—Cake, chocolate 0.4—Cake {others similar}— Cake icing, maximum value 0.5—candy (butterscotch 0.0—caramel 0.5— chocolate 0.5—Fudge 0.4—gum drops 0.0—peanut bars 0.9)—carrots (raw 9.0—boiled 7.2—canned, with liquid 4.3—canned, drained 4.0)—Cashew nuts 0.8—Cauliflower, raw 10.9—Cauliflower, frozen 10.2—Celery, raw 20.0—Celery, boiled 17.0—Chard, Swiss 22.0—Chard, Swiss, boiled 18.0—CHEESE (camembert 0.4—cheddar, American 0.3—cottage 0.8— cream 0.2—Swiss 0.3—pasteurized 0.2)—Cherries, sour 3.3—Cherries, sweet 2.7—Chestnuts 2.3—Chicken, light meat, roasted, no skin 2.5— Chicken, dark meat, roasted, no skin 1.8—Chives 8.9—Chop suey, canned 2.2—Clams 3.9—Coconut, dried 0.9—Coconut water 7.0—Cod, broiled 2.4—Coffee, instant 36.0—Collards 10.0—Collards, frozen 8.0—Corn, raw 3.0—Corn, boiled 2.0—Corn, canned, liquid 1.5—Corn, frozen 2.5— Corn grits, degreased 0.2—Corn flakes 0.3—Corn starch 0.0—Crab, canned 1.1—Cranberry 2.0—Cranberry sauce 0.2—Cream, half & half 1.0—Cream, heavy whipping 0.3—Cress 18.9—Cucumber 11.0 {also see pickels}— Custard, baked 1.3—Dandelion 8.8—Dates 2.4—Duck meat 1.7—Egg, frozen 0.8—Egg white, frozen 2.8—Egg yolk, frozen 0.3—Egg unfrozen, probably the same as frozen—Eggplant 8.5—Elderberries 4.2—Endive 14.7—Farina 0.2—Figs 2.3—Filberts 1.1—Flounder 2.9—Gelatin 0.0 {not from Handbook #8}—Gin 0.0—Goose, roasted meat 2.6—Grapefruit juice 4.2—Grapes, American 2.3—Grape juice canned 1.8—Grape juice, frozen 0.6—Grape juice, drink 0.6—Haddock, raw 3.8—Haddock, fried 2.1— Halibut, raw 4.5—Halibut, broiled 3.1—Herring, Pacific, raw 4.2—heart cooked (beef, lean—chicken 0.8—hog 0.7)—Honey 0.2—Horseradish, raw 6.5—Ice cream 0.4 to 0.9—Jams 0.3—Jelly 0.3—Jujube {Chinese date} 2.6— Kale, leaves 7.1—Kidneys, beef, cooked 1.3—Kohlrabi, raw 12.8—Lamb, 21% fat, raw 1.1—Lamb, 21% fat, cooked 0.9—Lard 0.0—Lemon juice, raw 5.5—Lentils 2.3—Lettuce, crisphead 13.4—Lettuce, looseleaf 14.7—Liver, beef, cooked 1.7—Liver, chicken, cooked 1.7—Lobster & shrimp, raw 2.4— Lobster, cooked & canned 1.9—Loganberries 3.1—Lychees 2.7—Macaroni, enriched 0.5—Milk 2.2—Milk, skimmed 4.0—Milk, human 0.7—Milk, goat 2.6—Molasses, light 3.6—Molasses, blackstrap 13.7—Mullet 2.0— Mushrooms 14.7—Muskmellon 8.4—muskmellon, frozen in syrup 3.0— Oatmeal 0.9—Ocean perch 4.1—Oils, salad or cooking 0.0—Okra, raw

6.9—Okra, boiled & drained 6.0—Okra, frozen 5.6—Okra, frozen, then boiled 4.3—Olives, green, pickled 0.5—Olives, ripe, pickled 0.3—Onions 4.1—Onions, boiled & drained 3.8—Onion tops 8.6—Orange juice 4.4—Orange drink, 40% 1.9—Oysters 1.8—Papayas 6.0—Parsley 16.5—Parsnips 7.1—Peaches 5.3—Peach nectar 1.6—Peanuts, roasted 1.2—Peanut butter, moderate added fat, salt, sweet1.0—Pears 2.1—PEAS (raw 3.8—canned, less liquid 1.1—frozen 2.1—split 2.6—boiled 2.8—edible pod 3.2)—Pecans 0.9—peppers, garden type 9.7—peppers, hot, pods 3.8—Perch, yellow 2.5—Persimmons 2.3—Pickles, dill 18.2 {sodium=130}—Pike, walleye 3.4—pineapple, raw 2.8—pineapple juice 2.7—Pistachio nuts 1.6—plums, raw 4.6—Pollack, raw 3.7—Pomegranite pulp, raw 4.1—Porgy & scup, raw 2.6—Pompano raw 1.2—Pork, ham, 28% fat, cooked 1.0—Pork, ham, 28% fat, raw 0.9—Pork, ham, cured, canned 1.8—Potatoes, raw 5.4—Potato chips 2.0—prickly pears 4.0—Prunes, uncooked 2.7—Prune juice 3.1—Pumpkin 13.0—Radishes 19.0—Raisins 2.7—RASPBERRIES (black, raw 2.7—red, raw 2.9—black, canned, with & without artificial sweetener 2.7—red, canned with & without artificial sweetener 3.3—red, frozen, sweetened 1.0)—Rhubarb 15.6—Rice, brown 0.6—Rice, white 0.3—Rice bran 5.4—Rice, flaked 0.5—Rice, puffed 0.3—Rockfish raw 4.0—Rockfish, oven cooked 4.2—Roe, cooked, baked, or boiled, cod & shad 1.0—Rutabaga, raw 5.2—Rutabaga, boiled 4.3—Rye, whole grain 1.4—Rye flour, light o.4—Rye flour, medium 0.6—Rye flour, dark 2.6—Sablefish, raw 1.9—salad dressing (mayonnaise 0.0—blue & roquefort 0.2—French 0.2—Italian 0.0—Russian 0.3—thousand island 0.2)—salmon, raw same as canned, some canned in brine (chinook, king 1.8—chum 2.4—coho, silver 2.2—pink, humpback 2.7—sockeye, red 1.9)— Sapodillas, raw 2.2—Sardines, Atlantic, canned in oil, drain 2.9—Sardines, Pacific canned in tomato sauce, solid & liquid 1.6—Sauerkraut, with liquid 7.8 {sodium=41.4}—Sausage 0.5-1.1—Scallops, cooked 4.3—seaweeds (Irish moss 1.3—kelp 2.1—wakame—1.1) (note: calories in sea weed may be undigestible)— Sesame seeds 1.3—Shrimp & lobster, raw 2.4—Sirup, cane 1.6—Sirup, maple 0.7—Sorghum grain, all 1.1—Soybeans, mature 4.3—Spaghetti, enriched 0.5—Spinach, raw 18.1—Spinach, boiled, drained 14.0—Spinach, frozen 17.0—Spinach, New Zealand 41.7—squash, raw (crookneck 10.1—Zucchini 11.9—acorn 8.7—butternut 9.0)—Strawberries, raw 4.4—Strawberries, frozen, sweetened 1.0—Sugar, brown 0.9—sugar, white 0.0—Sunflower seeds 1.6—Sweet potato 2.1—Sweet potato 2.1—Tamarinda, raw 3.3—Tangerine—2.8—Tangerine juice {fresh or canned}4.1—Tapioca 0.1—Taros, raw 5.2—Tartar sauce 0.1—Tea 12.5—tomatoes (raw 11.1—canned, low sodium 10.3—juice 12.0—catsup 3.4)— Tripe, beef 0.1—Tuna, canned in water, unsalted 2.2 Turkey flesh, roasted 1.9—Turnips 8.9—Turnip greens, canned 13.5—Veal, 15% fat, cooked—Vegetable juice 13.0—Vinegar 7.3—Walnuts 0.7—Watercress 14.8—Watermellon 3.8— wheat (whole grain 1.1—flour, whole 1.1—flour, white 0.3—bran 5.3—germ 2.3—puffed 0.9—puffed, & sugar—shredded 1.0) Whitefish, lake 1.9—Wine 1.1—Yeast, brewers 6.7—Yeast, bakers 7.1—Yoghurt, from skim 2.9—Yoghurt, from whole 2.1

CHAPTER 14
POTASSIUM IN FOOD , DESCENDING
CONTENT, MG/ CALORIE

Spinach, New Zealand 41.7; Coffee, instant 36; Beet greens 23.7; Chard, Swiss 22; Celery, raw 20; Bamboo shoots, 19.8; Radishes 19; Cress 18.9; Pickles, dill (sodium = 130) 19.2; Spinach, raw 18.1; Chard, Swiss, boiled 18; Celery, boiled 17; Spinach, frozen 17; Parsley 16.5; Rhubarb 15.6; Watercress 14.8; Endive 14.7; Lettuce, loose leaf 14.7, Mushrooms 14.7; Spinach, boiled, drained 14; Molasses, blackstrap 13,7; Turnip greens, canned 13.5 Lettuce, crisp head 13; Kohlrabi, raw 13.4; Pumpkin 13; Vegetable juice 13; Tea 12.5; Broccoli, raw 12; Tomato juice 12; Squash, zucchini 11.9; Tomatoes raw 11.1; Cucumber 11; Cauliflower, raw 10.8; Asparagus, frozen, 10.4; tomatoes, canned 10.3; Cauliflower, frozen 10.2, Asparagus, raw, 10.1; squash, raw crookneck 10.1; Collards 10; peppers, garden type 9.7; Squash, raw crookneck 9.7; Beans, green, snap canned, liquid, 9.5; Asparagus, canned, solids & liquids, 9.2; Asparagus, boiled, 9.1; Brussels sprouts, frozen, 9.1; Cabbage, raw 9; Carrots raw. 9; Squash, butternut 9; Brussels sprouts, frozen, boiled 8.9; Chives 8.9; Turnips 8.9; Dandelion 9.8; Broccoli, frozen 8.7; Brussels sprouts, raw 8.7; Squash, acorn 8.7; Onion tops 8.6; Broccoli, frozen, boiled 8.5; Eggplant 8.5; Cabbage, wedges, boiled 8.4; Musk melon 8.4; Cabbage, shredded, boiled, little water 8.1; Collards, frozen 8; Beets, raw 7.8; Sauerkraut, with liquid {sodium=41.4} 7.8; Beans, green, snap, raw 7.6; Vinegar 7.3; Carrots, boiled 7.2; Kale, leaves 7.1; Parsnips 7.1; Yeast, bakers 7.1; Coconut water 7; Okra, raw 6.9; Yeast, brewers 6.7; Apricots, canned, no sugar 6.5; Beets, cooked 6.5; Horseradish, raw 6.5; Beans, green, snap, frozen 6'4; Beans, mung, sprouted 6.4; Baby foods, beets, canned; 6.2; Beans, green, snap boiled, long time much water 6; Beans, green snap, boiled, short time, minimum water

6; Okra, boiled & drained 6; Papayas 6;Beans, green, snap, canned, low sodium with liquid 5.9; Beans, sprouted, mung, boiled 5.6; Okra, frozen 5.6; Apricots, raw 5.5; Lemon juice, raw 5.5; Baby foods tomato soup 5.4; Potatoes, raw 5.4; Rice bran 5.4; Beans, green, snap, canned, with liquid 5.3; Beans, lima, raw 5.3 Peaches 5.3; Wheat bran 5.3; Rutabaga, raw 5.2; Taros, raw 5.2; Beets, canned, & liquid 4.9; Beans, lima, frozen 4.8; plums, raw 4.6 Halibut, raw 4.5; bananas 4.4; Orange juice 4.4; Strawberries, raw 4.4; Carrrots, canned, with liquid 4.3; Okra, frozen, then boiled 4.3; Rutabaga, boiled 4.3; Scallops, cooked 4.3; Soybeans, mature 4.3; Baby foods, beans, green, caned 4.2; Elderberries 4.2; Grapefruit juice 4.2; Herring, Pacific, raw 4.2; Rockfish, oven cooked 4.2; Ocean perch 4.1; Onions 4.1; Pomegranite pulp, raw 4.1; Tangerine juice {fresh or canned) 4.1; Beans, green, snap, canned, solids only 4; Carrots, canned, drained 4; Milk, skimmed 4; prickly pears 4; Rockfish raw 4; Buttermilk 3.9; Clams 3.9; Beans, lima. Boiled 3.8; Haddock, raw 3.8; Onions, boiled & drained 3.8; Peas, raw 3.8; peppers, hot, pods 3.8; Water melon 3.8; Pollack, raw 3.7; Avocados 3.6; Beans, lima, frozen, baby 3.6; Molasses, light 3.6; Bean seeds, white, raw 3.5; Pike, walleye 3.4; Tomato catsup 3.4; Cherries, sour 3.3; Raspberries, red, canned, with & without artificial sweetener 3.3; Tamarinda, raw 3.3; Peas, edible pod 3.2; Beans, lima, canned & liquid 3.1; Halibut, broiled 3.1; Loganberries 3.1; Prune juice 3.1; Baby foods, cereal, high protein 3; Bran flakes 3; Corn, raw 3; musk mellon, frozen in syrup 3; Bean seeds, red, raw 2.9; Blackberries 2.9; Flounder 2.9; Sardines, Atlantic, canned in oil, drain 2.9; Yoghurt, from skim 2.9; Bass, sea 2.8; Egg white, frozen 2.8; Peas boiled 2.8; pineapple, raw 2.8; Tangerine 2.8; Apricot nectar 2.7; Cherries, sweet 2.7; Lychees 2.7; Pineapple juice 2.7; Prunes, uncooked 2.7; Raspberries, black, canned, with & without artificial sweetener 2.7; Raspberries, black, raw 2.7; Salmon, pink humpback 2.7; Beef, hamburger, lean 2.6; Goose, roasted meat 2.6; Jujube {Chinese date} 2.6; Milk, goat 2.6; Peas, split 2.6; Porgy & scup, raw 2.6; Rye flour, dark 2.6; Chicken, light meat, roasted, no skin 2.5; Corn, frozen 2.5; Perch, yellow 2.5, Cod, broiled 2.4; Dates 2.4; Lobster & shrimp, raw 2.4; Salmon chum 2.4; Apricots, frozen, sweetened 2.3; Beans, lima, canned, drained 2.3; Chestnuts 2.3; Figs 2.3; Grapes, American 2.3; Lentils 2.3; Persimmons 2.3; Wheat germ 2.3; Chop suey, canned 2.2; Milk 2.2; Salmon, coho, silver 2.2; Sapodillas, raw 2.2; Tuna, canned in water, unsalted 2.2; Apple juice 2.1; Haddock, fried 2.1; Pears 2.1; Peas, frozen 2.1; Pears 2.1; Sea weeds, kelp 2.1; Sweet potato 2.1; Yoghurt, from whole milk 2.1; Corn, boiled 2; Cranberry 2; Mullet 2; Potato chips 2; Apple 1.9; Baby foods, dinner, vegetable & bacon 1.9; Lobster, cooked & canned 1.9 Orange drink 1.9; Sablefish, raw 1.9; Salmon, raw same as canned, some canned in brine chinook, king 1.9; Turkey flesh, roasted 1.9; Whitefish, lake 1.9; Bacon, Canadian, fried 1.8; Bread, pumpernickel 1.8; Buckwheat, whole 1.8; Chicken, dark meat, roasted, no skin 1.8; Grape juice canned 1.8; Oysters 1.8; Pork, ham, cured, canned 1.8; Duck meat 1.7; Liver, beef or chicken, cooked 1.7; Beef, hamburger, regular 1.6; Brains, all kinds 1.6; Peach nectar 1.6; Pistachio nuts 1.6; Sardines, Pacific canned in tomato sauce, solid & liquid 1.6; Sirup, cane 1.6; Sunflower seeds 1.6; Blueberries, frozen 1.5; Corn, canned, liquid 1.5; Apple butter 1.5; Baby foods, banana and tapioca 1.4; Rye, whole grain 1.4; Almonds 1.3; Blueberries, raw 1.3; Custard, baked baked 1.3; Kidneys, beef, cooked 1.3; Sea weeds, Irish moss 1.3; Sesame seeds 1.3; Peanuts, roasted 1.2; Pompano raw 1.2; Beef, broiled or roasted, 18% fat 1.1; Brazil nuts 1.1; Crab, canned .1.1; Filberts 1.1; Lamb, 21% fat 1.1; Peas, canned, less liquid 1.1; Sea weeds, wakame 1.1; Sorghum grain, all 1.1; Wheat flour or grain whole 1.1; Wine 1.1; Cream, half % half 1; Peanut butter, moderate added fat, salt, sweet 1; Pork, ham, 28% fat, cooked 1; Roe, cooked, baked, or boiled, cod & shad 1; Baby foods, apple sauce 0.9; Baby foods, custard pudding 0.9; Candy, pea nut bar 0.9; Coconut, dried 0.9; Ice cream 0.9; Lamb, 21% fat, cooked 0.9; Oat meal 0.9; Pecans 0.9; Pork, ham, 28% fat, raw 0.9; Sugar, brown 0.9; Wheat, puffed 0.9; Baby foods fruit pudding 0.8; Blueberries, canned 0.8; Bouillion cubes {sodium=200.0} 0.8; Cashew nuts 0.8; Cheese, cottage 0.8; Heart chicken, cooked 0.8; Sausage 0.8; Heart, cooked 0.7; Milk, human 0.7; Syrup, maple 0.7; Walnuts 0.7; Beer 0.6; Blueberries, frozen with syrup 0.6; Bread, rye 0.6; Grape juice drink or frozen 0.6; Rice, brown 0.6; Barley 0.6; Bread, cracked wheat 0.5; Candy, caramel 0.5; Candy, chocolate 0.5; Macaroni, enriched 0,5; Olives, green, pickled 0.5; Spaghetti, enriched 0.5; Bacon, fried 0.4; BEEF, corned, medium fat 0.4; Blueberries, canned with syrup 0.4; Bread, white, 6% dry milk 0.4; Cake 0.4; Candy, fudge, 0.4; Cheese, camembert 0.4; Rye flour, light o.4; Cake, angel food 0.3; Cheese, cheddar 0.3; Cheese, Swiss 0.3; Corn flakes 0.3; Cream, heavy whipping 0,3; Egg yolk, frozen 0.3; Jams 0.3; Jelly 0,3; Olives, ripe, pickled 0.3; Rice, puffed or white 0.3; wheat flour, white 0.3; Cheese, cream 0.2, Corn grits, degreased 0.2; Cranberry sauce 0.2; Farina 0.2; Honey 0.2; Salad dressing, blue, Roquefort, thousand island, and French 0.2; Tapioca 0.1; Tartar sauce 0.1; Tripe, beef 0.1; Butter 0; Candy, butterscotch or gum drops 0; Oils, salad or cooking 0; Lard 0; Salad dressing, mayonnaise or Italian 0; Sugar, white 0.

CHAPTER 15
POPULAR HIGH POTASSIUM DIETS

By now hopefully you have been convinced of the importance of obtaining a healthy dose of potassium in your diet through the increased consumption of fruits and especially vegetables. Knowledge is power and the beginning of change is to desire it. But many studies show that in practice education about healthy dietary choices is not enough to get people to change their dietary habits.

There have been many public initiatives to increase fruit and vegetable consumption in order to promote health, reduce the risk of chronic diseases, and reduce the prevalence of overweight and obesity. Since 1916, the United States Department of Agriculture (USDA) has periodically issued Dietary Guidelines. In 1956 it recommended eating according to Four Basic Food Groups. Most Americans are aware of the "5 a day" program, initiated in 1991 by the National Cancer Institute, which was aimed at increasing increasing fruit and vegetable consumption since numerous controlled studies link diets rich in fruits and vegetables with a decreased risk of many health problems. In 1992, the Four Basic Food Groups became a Food Pyramid which now recommends 8-10 servings of fruits and vegetables a day. In 1994 the Nutrition Labeling and Education Act required labeling on food to allow the public to more easily follow the Food Guide Pyramid. Both the Dietary Guidelines for Americans and the My Pyramid Food Guidance System, which translates nutritional recommendations into the kinds and amounts of food to eat each day, are available at [http://www.cnpp.usda.gov/]. Many aides to help the public follow these recommendations can be found at that site.

In addition to specific food group and nutrient recommendations, the 2010 Dietary Guidelines also mentions three diets which studies have linked to reduced risk of chronic disease: the DASH diet (Dietary Approaches to Stop Hypertension), the Mediterranean Diet, and Vegetarian-style diets.

Studies show promising results for other diets but the USDA says they do not know enough about these diets to include them.

The 2010 Dietary Guidelines lists potassium, calcium, Vitamin D, and fiber, (and, in pregnant women, folate, B12, and iron) as 'nutrients of concern' which are significantly under consumed in the American diet Of course "fiber" is not a nutrient. The average American diet contains only 3 fruits and vegetables of the recommended 9-10 per day and 2,750 (or less in some states and much less for black people) of the daily 4,700 mg of the potassium the Dietary Guidelines recommends for health. Some of the shortfall comes due to poor estimation of portion sizes. A USDA study in 2000 entitled, "Consumption of Food Group Servings: People's Perceptions vs. Reality" revealed actual fruit and vegetable intake was only 60-75% of estimated intake on food logs kept by study subjects.

Although the Dietary Guidelines list fruits, vegetables, and low fat dairy products as good sources of potassium (dairy products are only fair sources), the potassium that is obtained in the American diet comes from poor sources. According to the National Health and Nutrition Examination Survey (NHANES) 2005–06, the five most common sources of potassium in the average American diet are reduced fat milk (154 mg/day), coffee (135 mg/day), chicken and chicken mixed dishes (119 mg/day), beef and beef mixed dishes (94 mg/day), and 100% orange/grapefruit juice (90 mg/day). http://riskfactor.cancer.gov/diet/foodsources/potassium/.

According to NHANES III (2004), the median intakes of sodium among adult men and women are 4,300 mg and 2,900 mg of sodium per day, respectively, which is too high for health.

Potassium is freely available in a wide variety of foods but unfortunately, it is easily lost in cooking. As much as 50% can be lost when food is boiled. Steaming gives better results, although an appreciable amount is still leached into the water. It's far better, where possible, to eat foods raw or to make them into soups where the cooking water can be used. Either that, or use the boil water. Alcohol, coffee and other caffeine drinks, sugar and diuretic drugs cause further potassium losses.

I would like to highlight 5 diets high in potassium below:

1. DASH diet

2. Ph Balance Diet / Vermont Folk Medicine

3. Macrobiotic Diet

4. Gerson Diet

5. Vegetarian Diet

The first four of these diets have as their goal increasing intake of fruits and vegetables in order to increase potassium for health, whereas the 5th diet is generally undertaken for moral or religious reasons, yet as a byproduct increases fruit and vegetable consumption and is usually also associated with health benefits. It does not necessarily remove low potassium foods such as whole wheat, though. Let's take briefly a look at each of these high potassium diets.

DASH DIET

The DASH diet (Dietary Approaches to Stop Hypertension) is clinically proven to significantly lower hypertension. It features foods known to be high in potassium, calcium, and magnesium, and low in sodium. According to the NIH (National Institutes of Health), the DASH diet targets a daily dose of 4,700 mg of potassium and 1500-2300 mg of sodium. Although there is current evidence that hypertension is related to the chloride present in salt, limiting sodium consumption per DASH guidelines has been proven effective probably because all chloride is associated with sodium except sodium bicarbonate in pastries, for which you should substitute potassium bicarbonate.

The DASH diet in a Nutshell:

Vegetables	4-5 servings / day (this would be better higher)
Fruits	4-5 servings / day
Low fat milk	2-3 servings / day
Grains	6-8 servings / day (this should be lower)
Meats/fish	6 oz. or less / day (more is better, at each meal)
Nuts, seeds, legumes	4-5 servings / week
Fats / oils	2-3 ts. / day (oils should be unsaturated)
Sweets/sugars	5 Tbs./week or less (preferably as molasses)
Sodium	1500-2300 milligrams / day

NOTE: Although dehydration thickens blood, which increases blood pressure, the DASH diet is silent on fluid intake, indicating the thirst mechanism is sufficient to ensure adequate hydration. This is not always true and some dietitians instruct their hypertensive patients with healthy kidneys to consume 8 glasses of unsweetened, uncaffeinated fluid/day.

WHERE IS THE POTASSIUM? WHERE IS THE SALT

In practice, people do not usually know where the potassium or sodium is in their diets, nor which food processing and preparation methods best maintain potassium. People assume they eat a low salt diet if they leave the salt shaker alone, but they are not conscious of the amount of sodium already present in various foodstuffs, nor are they aware that on the order of 75% of potassium can be lost from a food in its raw state through processing and preparation by the time it winds up on the plate. For someone who never eats out, leaves the salt shaker alone, and eats as many of his/her fruits and vegetables raw as possible, the DASH diet as a simple rule of thumb may work.

Most people learning the diet are going to have to spend 2 weeks writing down every single thing they eat and drink and making daily tallies of their potassium and sodium intakes. After 2 weeks they will probably have learned to make dietary choices that meet DASH potassium and sodium goals, they will know by heart the potassium and sodium content of their favorite foods if they access table 13 or 14 of this book, and they will be able to estimate sodium content in broad classes of foods and the relative potassium loss effects of various food processing and preparation methods.

To start, give yourself a budget of 500 mg sodium per meal and 300 milligrams per day for snacks. Do not target the higher limit of sodium allowed as miscalculations will occur. To make it easy on yourself and encourage potassium consumption, don't count sodium present in raw fruits and vegetables but do count any present in canned or prepared fruits and vegetables, or better yet do not eat canned food. This will enable you to make realistic choices and, for example, budget out that piece of processed "cheese food" that doesn't add much to your sandwich and that bagel. Bread and some dairy products contain a lot of salt, so should not be eaten. You should choose foods in the least processed form available, such as choosing a baked potato over french fries and cole slaw and chicken salad without mayonnaise (mayonnaise is high in salt and fat).

When eating out, pass on casseroles and stick to basic foods whose salt content you can estimate. The salt is usually found in the sauces, gravies, cheeses, butters, margarines, spreads, condiments, dressings, toppings, breadings, and soups. Read the menu carefully. Words like spicy, basted, or marinaded, usually indicate added salt. Many restaurants have a list of the salt content of their meals for those with dietary challenges. Ask for it. Better yet, stay out of restaurants. Asian cuisines such as Thai, Chinese, and Japanese, are known to be extremely high in sodium.

Often even the vegetable choices will be high in sodium chloride, and it may not be possible to find acceptable food choices on their menus. Italian restaurants feature sodium chloride loaded bread and cheese dishes, and often rely on high-sodium chloride canned tomato products for their sauces. Spicy dishes, such as found in Mexican cuisines, are usually high in sodium chloride, and refried beans often come from cans pre-salted.

If you have high blood pressure, there is no substitute for tracking it daily. When learning the diet or introducing new foods it is important to measure blood pressure before and after meals to find out how your food choices affect you. Fruit juice can also raise blood sugar. Sweets also spike up the blood sugar which crashes later. 1960's nutritionist Adele Davis wrote that low blood sugar causes a loss of so much potassium that it takes 6 bananas to replace it.

Herbs are high in potassium, such as sage, parsley, rosemary, basil, dill, and mint. Hops and red clover are high in both potassium and phytoestrogens. Try replacing salt with herbs in your cooking and experiment with herbal teas. 1 tablespoon of mint herbal tea has 8 mg of potassium. 1 tablespoon burdock, which makes a pleasant tea, contains 23 mg of potassium. A surprise source of potassium is blackstrap molasses: 1 tablespoon has 600 mg.

DASH does not point out that salt is the main source of iodide in many regions, so any salt reduction diet must include iodide (but not iodate) supplementation. Indeed, people do not get as much iodide as would be the most optimum for health anyway from salt, and supplements are in order with any diet.

DASH is a Cornerstone. Depending on how high your blood pressure is, you may need to employ additional measures (such as methylfolate, calcium, magnesium, arginine, garlic, celery, chocolate, and/or medications, to name a few) to lower your blood pressure sufficiently for health. However experience says that no dietary measure short of correcting your potassium and sodium intakes and ratio will succeed. Should medication be necessary, following DASH recommendations and advice in this book will reduce the amount of medication needed.

VERMONT FOLK MEDICINE

Throughout the centuries there have been healers who have interpreted and systematized the folk medicine that arises from people's observation of nature and animals. Dr. D.C. Jarvis, a Vermont country doctor, studied the folk medicine of rural Vermont in humans and livestock, broke it down into basic principles, and documented them in his 1958 classic, "Folk Medicine", which is still in print today. Dr. Jarvis observed the diet that brought health was high-carbohydrate, low-protein, and acid in reaction before it enters the mouth, sour tasting (This may have been helpful because hydrogen ion interferes with potassium excretion). In particular a diet full of raw food: berries, fruits, leaves, and roots (it would not have had to be raw if they realized the losses from boiling), A common folk remedy was to drink a teaspoon of apple cider vinegar in a glass of water upon rising. Dr. Jarvis reasoned that by so doing farmers were achieving acid/alkaline balance which could be measured by testing their urine with litmus paper. He performed many studies on humans and livestock which showed that cider vinegar helped one avoid illness. Experimenting with other vinegars showed no other would produce the same result, which he attributed to the potassium in combination with other minerals from the apple. One of his studies involved 24 people who were instructed to record their urinary pH in conjunction with various data for two years. Dr. Jarvis met with them on a regular basis to go over their records. He found that 2 days before they became sick, their urinary pH would become alkaline. He found that the apple cider vinegar mixture could be used to keep the urine acidic and thus avert the illness or render it mild. From this study he found the following things cause an alkaline urine:

1. Incipient illness

2. Stress

3. Sleeping with a window open in cold weather (whereas a hot bath would shift urine back to acid)

4. Physical and mental fatigue

5. Pain (sinusitis, arthritis, neuralgia)

6. Certain foods: wheat, sugar, many others

7. Whereas sour foods would acidify the urine

Dr. Jarvis observed that when healthy foods were available, children instinctively chose those best for them (if only nutritious food was placed before those children, they could hardly have missed). Adults seemed to have lost that ability in his view. He proposed that we adults could use the urine reaction to substitute for our discarded instincts (there is little chance that such an instinct exists).

Dr. Jarvis requested a colleague on the faculty of a medical school to prepare for him a list of bacteria harmful to the human body together with the pH of the media most favorable for their growth. He published the list, which included staph, strep, pneumonia, influenza influenza is a virus, and others, all of which grow in an alkaline media. By correcting the acid/alkaline balance of the body, Dr. Jarvis found it possible to fend off all manner of illnesses in his practice, rendering it unnecessary to bother diagnosing the precise infection. He found that the amount of apple cider vinegar to add to a glass of water depended on the individual and could be governed by the amount of sourness that tasted good to them.

When corn is grown in potassium-poor soil, a reddish precipitate forms on the nodes of the joints that shuts off the circulation of the sap from the root to the leaves. Analysis of this precipitate indicates it is composed of iron. Conversely when potassium is added to the soil, no iron is precipitated to block the sap channels. Dr. Jarvis questioned whether or not the lymph channels in people and animals could become similarly blocked (there is virtually no chance that there could be a similar mechanism in animals). He observed in clinical practice that enlarged lymph nodes could be cleared when potassium was supplied to the body. Through various means, Dr. Jarvis discovered that potassium controls the use of calcium in the body. He found that broken bones that would not knit could be made to do so by taking 1 kelp tablet per meal as a source of potassium (One kelp tablet will not furnish much potassium or calcium. So something else was happening). Dr. Jarvis advised that people take in twice the amount of potassium, in the form of fresh vegetables, fruits, and berries, as the amount of sodium. He said the older you grow the greater should be your daily intake of potassium. Some easy ways he listed to increase potassium are through the use of paprika, apple cider vinegar and honey in a glass of water, kelp, and grape, apple, or cranberry juice (he was mistaken about honey). It must be remembered that many farmers of 1958 would be what are called organic farmers today. For example, there is 18% more potassium in organic produce than non-organic according to nutritional value of crops as influenced by organic and inorganic fertilizer treatments and other nutrients show an even greater advantage — Results of 12 years' experiments with vegetables (1960–1972), W. Schuphan, Plant Foods for Human Nutrition, vol 23, no. 4, 333-358. [http://www. springerlink.com/content/p45041417m45185q/]

MACROBIOTIC DIET

The Macrobiotic diet is an interpretation of Traditional Chinese Medicine that has existed for thousands of years. Healers universally observed that dietary balance is required for health, which is what we attempt with our Dietary Guidelines by which we group foods and teach selection of foods from each group and, further, selection of produce from each color. In Chinese medicine, the healers observed the same types of health problems in the same types of people and found that people who tended toward anemia and melancholy (which they called yin) could be helped by balancing their diets with more of the type of food eaten by people who tended toward a ruddy-complexion, irritability, and high blood pressure (which they called yang) and vice versa. They grouped foods that appeared tall, thin, dilute, and cool (the diet of the yin people) and called them "yin". They grouped foods that appeared short, round, dense, and warm (the diet of the yang people) and called them "yang". As you can expect, most foods do not fit neatly into those categories, and it became an art to judge the relative degree of yin or yang each food represents. Yin-yang eating does cause food selection by color since warm colors (red) are considered more yang in a continuum through cool colors (violet), which are yin. But there is more than color behind macrobiotics. Macrobiotics is an ancient diet concerned with mineral and acid-alkaline balance. Unfortunately for the yin-yang concept, there is no correlation at all between color or shape and nutrition, personality, or hypertension.

Thousands of years ago when the yin-yang concept developed there was no chemical periodic table, no microscope, and no litmus paper. In the late 1800's, Sagan Ishizuka, a Japanese army doctor who suffered from a kidney disease since the age of 5, found that the ying-yang diet helped him. At a time when modern medicine cared only about protein, carbohydrate, and fat, Dr. Ishizuka reached the idea that proper diet is all about balance of potassium and sodium in foods. He carried out many clinical trials and cured many people from serious health problems.

ORIGIN OF MACROBIOTIC WORD

In the 1920's, Japanese George Oshawa interpreted the traditional yin-yang principle as enriched by Dr. Ishizuka in the light of modern science and called it macrobiotics. He identified yang foods as alkaline and yin foods as acidic. His teachings can be confusing because yin is always in reference to yang. So although all vegetables are yin compared to a concentrated food like meat, carrots that grow under the ground are considered yang compared to fruit that grow high in a tree, which he viewed as very yin (however keep in mind that the altitude at which a food grows has no nutritional significance).

Oshawa classified the yin and yang of foods by potassium to sodium ratio (K to Na) and the difference between potassium and sodium content (K-Na). Oshawa set the ideal ratio of potassium to sodium in man's foods at 5:1, but that the ratio could fluctuate between 3:1 and 7:1 depending on his living environment. Individual foods with a potassium to sodium ratio of over 100 were considered very yin, foods with a potassium to sodium ratio of less than 10 were considered very yang, and those in between were well balanced. Oshawa classified the yin and yang of foods by potassium to sodium ratio (K to :Na) and the difference between potassium and sodium content

One of Oshawa's students, Herman Aihara, applied chemistry to the yin-yang principles in the manner of his teacher. He tested many foods for their relative acidity and mineral content, published lists, and boiled down rules of thumb in a pithy book on the subject. The classic book "Acid & Alkaline" by Herman Aihara is still in print today.).

HISTORY OF MACROBIOTIC DIET FROM YIN AND YANG

The Macrobiotic diet is an interpretation of Traditional Chinese Medicine that has existed for thousands of years. Healers universally assumed that dietary balance is required for health, which is what they attempted with Dietary Guidelines by which foods are grouped and selection of foods from each group is taught and, further, selection of produce from each color. In Chinese medicine, the healers observed the same types of health problems in the same types of people and found that people who tended toward anemia and melancholy (which they called yin) could be helped by balancing their diets with more of the type of food eaten by people who tended toward a ruddy-complexion, irritability, and high blood pressure (which they called yang) and vice versa. They grouped foods that appeared tall, thin, dilute, and cool (the diet of the yin people) and called them "yin". They grouped foods that appeared short, round, dense, and warm (the diet of the yang people) and called them "yang". As you can expect, most foods do not fit neatly into those categories, and it became an art to judge the relative degree of yin or yang each food represents. It must have given these ancient healers a lot of useless activity futilely attempting to make sense out of nonsense. Yin-yang eating does cause food selection by color since warm colors (red) are considered more yang in a continuum through cool colors (violet), which are yin. But there is more than color behind macrobiotics. Macrobiotics is an ancient diet concerned with mineral and acid-alkaline balance.

Thousands of years ago when the yin-yang concept developed there was no chemical periodic table, no microscope, and no litmus paper. In the late 1800's, Sagan Ishizuka, a Japanese army doctor who suffered from a kidney disease since the age of 5, found that the ying-yang diet helped him. At a time when modern medicine cared only about protein, carbohydrate, and fat, Dr. Ishizuka reached the idea that proper diet is all about balance of potassium and sodium in foods. He carried out many clinical trials and cured many people from serious health problems.

One of Oshawa's students, Herman Aihara, applied chemistry to the yin-yang principles in the manner of his teacher. He tested many foods for their relative acidity and mineral content, published lists, and boiled down rules of thumb in a pithy book on the subject. The classic book "Acid & Alkaline" by Herman Aihara is still in print today.

He explains the concept of acid-forming foods and alkaline-forming foods. These are foods that, regardless of their pH outside the body, become acid or alkaline upon digestion, for he assumed it is the mineral content of food which ultimately determines the acidity or alkalinity it will cause in the body. To determine whether a food is acid forming or alkaline forming, he proposed it must be burned to ashes (simulating digestion), added to a standard amount of pure water, then tested by determining how much of a known alkaline solution must be added to neutralize the acid, or vice versa. He said the relative acidity of a food could be approximated by its ratio of calcium to phosphorus. He summarized what he found in a simple list which can be used as a rule of thumb for macrobiotics:

- Yin Alkaline-forming foods. Fruits, vegetables, seeds, honey, coffee, herb tea, bancha tea. He said these foods tend to be high in potassium and calcium but not in phosphorus and sulfur (keep in mind that honey is not high in potassium).
- Yang Alkaline forming foods. Radish pickle, dry soy sauce, miso, salted umboshi, salt. He said these foods tend to be high in sodium and magnesium but not in phosphorus and sulfur.
- Yin Acid forming foods. Beans, nuts, chemical drugs, pills, sugar, candy, soft drinks, alcohol drinks. He said these foods tend to be high in phosphorus and sulfur but not in sodium.
- Yang Acid forming foods. Animal foods, grains. He said these foods tend to be high in phosphorus and sulfur and sodium (there is no resemblance of grain to meat in just about any respect).

Aihara classifies sweets, drugs, and all refined foods as acid forming because they are lacking in minerals, especially alkaline forming minerals. Therefore the body cannot neutralize the acid that is created by them without using mineral stores to do so (no acids are created by sugar or medicines, unless the medicine itself is acid, in which case the amounts are usually insignificant)).

In Macrobiotics, he said balance must be achieved by selecting foods from these groups (and further, selecting foods within each group that are closest to pH neutral, for macrobiotics teaches that trying to balance strongly acidic and alkaline foods is precarious and not likely to succeed.

He explained the concept of acid-forming foods and alkaline-forming foods. These are foods that, regardless of their pH outside the body, become acid or alkaline upon digestion, for it is the mineral content of food which ultimately determines the acidity or alkalinity it will cause in the body. To determine whether a food is acid forming or alkaline forming, it must be burned to ashes, simulating digestion, added to a standard amount of pure water, then tested by determining how much of a known alkaline solution must be added to neutralize the acid, or vice versa. He said the relative acidity of a food could be approximated by its ratio of calcium to phosphorus.

Aihara classified sweets, drugs, and all refined foods as acid forming, because they are lacking in minerals, especially alkaline forming minerals. Therefore the body cannot neutralize the acid that is created by them without using mineral stores to do so.

In Macrobiotics balance must be achieved by selecting foods from these groups, and further, selecting foods within each group that are closest to pH neutral, for macrobiotics teaches that trying to balance strongly acidic and alkaline foods is precarious and not likely to succeed.

The macrobiotic diet which has kept people healthy for thousands of years (as every diet consisting of unprocessed vegetables and meat has) contains many ethnic foods unheard of in the Western World. Changes in the diet, even according to established principles, is not guaranteed to work (there is very little in this world that can be guaranteed). It should be said that Macrobiotics has been both vindicated and reviled in the Western medical community, which classifies it as a vegetarian diet (in actual fact, the diet calls for fish several times a week). Many studies of vegetarian diets, in which study participants are chosen from amongst the macrobiotic community and others, have shown many health benefits. On the other hand, studies have ridiculed Macrobiotics as low in Vitamin D (this is a meaningless ridicule because ALL diets are low in vitamin D that do not contain liver).

Macrobiotics furnishes some epidemiological evidence that eating an unprocessed food diet is healthy, but not much other useful information. Those ancient nutritionists did the best they could, but they were groping in the dark. Having read this book, and with the aid of the tables, you will have no trouble getting all the potassium you need. Eat ONLY unprocessed food, supplement iodide and vitamin D and supplement potassium when some disaster or illness depletes your potassium (see chapter 8) and this will go a long way toward keeping you healthy and give you a long, productive life.

ABOUT THE AUTHOR

Charles Weber has been interested in scientific studies as long as he can remember his childhood.

He spent most of his high school years studying science and math. He attended one half of a year studying chemical engineering at Cooper Union. He spent the equivalent of a couple of years studying aviation and ordinance at Colgate University, Athens University. Kilgore College, and a series of marvelous Navy schools. He has one year of mechanical engineering at Rutgers University and 3 years of chemistry there. He has the equivalent of between one and two years studying soil science at Cook College, which earned him a master's degree in soil science.

He spent several years as an analytical chemist and then in the next position a year as a development chemist at which time they moved their research out west. Even this long ago he had objected to management lining cement-asbestos pipes with fluoride, which did not endear him to them. He made a living of from then on for most of the rest of his life as an electrician and excavating contractor.

However, he really pictures him self as a theorist. None of his hypotheses have been accepted by the scientific community, except his hypotheses concerning potassium and copper nutrition, and these only reluctantly and partially lately by the medical community. None have been invalidated though. He has spent most of his adult life studying potassium and copper nutrition as an avocation, and he probably knows more about those subjects than anyone in the world. He had written a book about the relation of potassium to rheumatoid arthritis several decades ago. He has published articles on allied subjects in; The Journal of Theoretical Biology (1970, 1983), The Journal of Applied Nutrition (1974) which gained the best article of the year award, Clinical and Experimental Rheumatology (1983), and Medical Hypotheses (1984, 1999, 2007, 2008).

The information in this book is based almost entirely on solid scientific experimental evidence or epidemiological studies. The only exceptions are a few individual case histories and a few private communications.

In any case, He wishes you all good health, and he is certain that this book will enable you to be much healthier.

The author would like to thank Dr. Reza Rastmanesh for helpful suggestions and for testing potassium against rheumatoid arthritis, Steven Weber for proof reading some chapters, Susan Wolcott for much information and for writing most of chapter 15, Katherine Poehlmann for suggestions, Lee Armstrong for the cover design, Tom Czirok for editing the cover, Kacy Czirok for archiving the material, and all of the author's immediate family for all kinds of indirect assistance.

REFERENCES

References are presented as they occur in each chapter.

INTRODUCTION

Blundell JE Green S. & Barley VJ 1994 Carbohydrates and human appetite. American Journal of Clinical Nutrition 59 (suppl) ; 728 s-734 s.

Darrow DC & Pratt EL 1951 Handbook of Nutrition - 2nd edition p482-487. Blakiston Co., NY

Forman R. 1981 Medical resistance to innovation. Med Hypotheses. 7(8):1009-17.

Hadhazy VA Ezzo J Creamer P Berman BM 2000 Mind - body therapies for the treatment of fibromyalgia, a systematic review. Journal Rheumatol. 27;2911-2918.

Jentoft ES Kvalik AG Mengshoel AM 2001 Effects of pool - based and land based aerobic exercise on women with fibromyalgia / chronic widespread pain. Arthritis Rheum. 45; 42-47.

Oliver WJ Cohen EL Neel JV 1975 Blood pressure, sodium intake, and sodium related hormones in the Yanomamo Indians "no salt culture". Circulation 52;146151.

Saltin B Astrand P-O 1993 Free fatty acids and exercise. American Journal of Clinical Nutrition 57 (suppl) 752 s-758 s.

Scribner BH & Burnell JM 1956 . Metabolism 5; 468-479.

Weber CE 1974 Potassium in the etiology of rheumatoid arthritis and heart infarction. Journal of Applied Nutrition 26; 41-67.

Westerterp KR 1993 Food quotient, respiratory quotient, and energy balance.
American Journal of Clinical Nutrition 57(suppl); 759 s-765 s.

CHAPTER 1; POTASSIUM IN FOOD

Chan JM, Stampfer MJ, Ma J, Gann PH, Gaziano JM, Giovannucci EL. 2001 Dairy products, calcium, and prostate cancer risk in the Physicians' Health Study. Am J Clin Nutr 74(4):549-54.

Dahl, et al 1972 Influence of dietary potassium and sodium/ potassium molar ratios on the development of salt hypertension. Journal of Experimental Medicine 136; 318-330.

Funahashi, H., Imaj, T., Tanaka, Y., et al, 1996 Suppressive Effect of Iodine on DMBA-Induced Breast Tumor Growth in the Rat, Journal of Surgical Oncology, 61; 209-213,

Grace ND O'Dell BL 1970 Effect of magnesium deficiency on the distribution of water and cations in the muscle of the guinea pig. J. Nutr. 100; 45-50.

Hadhazy VA Ezzo J Creamer P Berman BM 2000 Mind - body therapies for the treatment of fibromyalgia, a systematic review. Journal Rheumatol. 27;2911-2918.

Hu FB Stampfer MI Rimm EB Manson JE Aschiro A Colditz GA Rosner BA Spiegelman D Speizer FE Sacks FM Hennekens CH Willett WC 1999 A prospective study of egg consumption and risk of cardiovascular disease in men and women. JAMA 281 (15); 1387-1394.

Jentoft ES Kvalik AG Mengshoel AM 2001 Effects of pool - based and land based aerobic exercise on women with fibromyalgia / chronic widespread pain. Arthritis Rheum. 45; 42-47.

Liu PT Stenger S Li H Wenzel L Tan BH Krutzik SR Ochoa MT Schauber J Wu K Meinken C Kamen DL Wagner M Bals R Steinmeyer Zugel U Gallo RL Eisenberg D Hewison M Hollis BW Adams JS Bloom BR Modlin RL 2006 Toll-like receptor triggering of a vitamin D-mediated human antimicrobial response. Science 311; 1770-1773.

Mann GV 1977 Diet-Heart: end of an era. New England Journal of Medicine 297; 644-650.

Nagataki S, Shizume K, and Nakao K. 1967 Thyroid function in chronic excess iodide ingestion: Comparison of thyroidal absolute iodine uptake and degradation of thyroxine in euthyroid Japanese subjects. J Clin Endo, 27; 638-647.

Oliver WJ Cohen EL Neel JV 1975 Blood pressure, sodium intake, and sodium related hormones in the Yanomamo Indians "no salt culture". Circulation 52;146-151.

Perez-Guzman C Vargas MH Quinonez F Bazavilvazo N Aguilar A 2005 A Cholesterol-Rich Diet Accelerates Bacteriologic Sterilization in Pulmonary Tuberculosis. Chest. 2005;127:643-651.

Rauma A-L Torronen R Hanninen O Mykkanen H 1995 ViaminB-12 status of long term adherents of a strict uncooked vegan diet ("living food") diet is compromised. Journal of Nutrition 125;2511-2515. Comments by Davis DR et al in the 1997 issue, start p378.

Saltin B Astrand P-O 1993 Free fatty acids and exercise. American Journal of Clinical Nutrition 57 (suppl) 752 s-758 s.

Slater G, et. al., Nutrition Reports International, vol. 14 (1976), page 249.

Stadel B. 1976 Dietary iodine and risk of breast, endometrial, and ovarian cancer. The Lancet, 1;890-891.

Stehbens WE 2004 Hypothetical hypercholesterolemia and atherosclerosis. Medical Hypotheses 62; 72-78.

Weber CE 1974 Potassium in the etiology of rheumatoid arthritis and heart infarction. Journal of Applied Nutrition 26; Nos 1&2, 41-67.(bibliography must be acquired separately).

CHAPTER 2: OTHER NUTRIENTS IN FOOD

Aremu DA Madejczyk MS Balletori N 2008 N-acetylcysteine as a potential antidote and biomonitoring agent of methylmercury exposure. Environmental Health Perspectives. 116; 26-31.

Chan JM, Stampfer MJ, Ma J, Gann PH, Gaziano JM, Giovannucci EL. 2001 Dairy products, calcium, and prostate cancer risk in the Physicians' Health Study. American Journal of Clinical Nutrition 74(4):549-54.

Dahl, et al 1972 Influence of dietary potassium and sodium/ potassium molar ratios on the development of salt hypertension. Journal Experimental Medicine 136; 318-330.

Doyle R 2002 Down on the farm. Scientific American 287 No2; 27.

Funahashi H Imaj T Tanaka Y, et al, 1996 Suppressive Effect of Iodine on DMBA-Induced Breast Tumor Growth in the Rat, Journal of Surgical Oncology, 61; 209-213,

Grace ND O'Dell BL 1970 Effect of magnesium deficiency on the distribution of water and cations in the muscle of the guinea pig. Journal of Nutrition 100; 45-50.

Griffith RS, DeLong DC, Nelson JD 1981 Relation of arginine-lysine antagonism to herpes simplex growth in tissue culture. Chemotherapy ;27(3):209-13.

Hadhazy VA Ezzo J Creamer P Berman BM 2000 Mind - body therapies for the treatment of fibromyalgia, a systematic review. Journal Rheumatol. 27;2911-2918.

Hu FB Stampfer MI Rimm EB Manson JE Aschiro A Colditz GA Rosner BA Spiegelman D Speizer FE Sacks FM Hennekens CH Willett WC 1999 A prospective study of egg consumption and risk of cardiovascular disease in men and women. JAMA 281 (15); 1387-1394.

Ivie GW Holt DL Ivey MG 1981 Natural toxicants in human foods: psoralans in raw and cooked parsnip root. Science 213 No. 4510 ; 909-910.

LaVecchia c Decarli A Pagano R 1998 Vegetable consumption and risk of chronic disease. Epidemiology 9; 208-210.

Le Marchand L, Kolonel LN, Nomura AM.1985 Breast cancer survival among Hawaiian Japanese and Caucasian women: ten-year rates and survival by place of birth.Am. J. of Epidemiol.;122:571-578.

Liu PT Stenger S Li H Wenzel L Tan BH Krutzik SR Ochoa MT Schauber J Wu K Meinken C Kamen DL Wagner M Bals R Steinmeyer Zugel U Gallo RL Eisenberg D Hewison M Hollis BW Adams JS Bloom BR Modlin RL 2006 Toll-like receptor triggering of a vitamin D-mediated human antimicrobial response. Science 311; 1770-1773.

Mann GV 1977 Diet-Heart: end of an era. New England J. of Medicine 297; 644-650.

McCune MA, Perry HO, Muller SA, O'Fallon WM 1984 Treatment of recurrent herpes simplex infections with L-lysine monohydrochloride. Cutis Oct;34(4):366-73.

Nagata C, Shimizu H. Risk factors for breast cancer 1996 Findings from comparative studies on Japanese in Japan, Japanese and whites in the United States. Gann Monograph on Cancer Research ;44:51-57.

Nagataki S, Shizume K, and Nakao K. 1967 Thyroid function in chronic excess iodide ingestion: Comparison of thyroidal absolute iodine uptake and degradation of thyroxine in euthyroid Japanese subjects. J Clin Endo, 27; 638 647.

Nikkels AF, Pierard GE.1994 Recognition and treatment of shingles. Drugs. Oct;48(4):528-48.

Pattison, D. 2004 Arthritis & Rheumatism, Vol 50: pp 3804-3812.

Perez-Guzman C Vargas MH Quinonez F Bazavilvazo N Aguilar A 2005 A Cholesterol-Rich Diet Accelerates Bacteriologic Sterilization in Pulmonary Tuberculosis. Chest. 2005;127:643-651.-

Rauma A-L Torronen R Hanninen O Mykkanen H 1995 ViaminB-12 status of long term adherents of a strict uncooked vegan diet ("living food") diet is compromised. Journal of Nutrition 125;2511-2515. Comments by Davis DR et al in the 1997 issue, start p378.

Slater G, et. al., 1997 Nutrition Reports International 14; 249.

Stadel B. 1976 Dietary iodine and risk of breast, endometrial, and ovarian cancer. The Lancet, 1;890-891.

Stehbens WE 2004 Hypothetical hypercholesterolemia and atherosclerosis. Medical Hypotheses 62; 72-78.

Tavera-Mendoza LE White JH 2007 Cell defenses and the sunshine vitamin. Scientific American 297; 62-72.

Uauy C Distelfeld A Fahima T Blecht A Dubcovky J 2006 A NAC gene regulating senescence improves grain protein, zinc, and iron content in wheat. Science 314;1298-1301.

Van Duyn MA Pivonka E 2000 Overview of the health benefits of fruit and vegetable consumption for the dietetics professional: selected literature. Journal of the American Dietetic Association. Dec;100(12):1511-21.

Weber CE 1984 Copper response in rheumatoid arthritis. Medical Hypotheses 15; 333-348.

Weber CE 2005 Eliminate infection (abscess) in teeth with cashew nuts. Medical Hypotheses 65; 1200.

Weber CE 2008 Does capsaicin in chili case diabetes. Medical Hypotheses 71 (2); 523-524.

Wilkinson RJ Llewelyn M Toosi Z et al 2000 Influence of vitamin D deficiency and vitamin D receptor polymorphisms on tuberculosis among Gyarati Asians in West London: a case controlled study. Lancet 355; 618-621.

CHAPTER 3: HEART DISEASE AND HYPERTENSION

Allen KGD & Klevay LM Copper deficiency and cholesterol metabolism in the rat. 1978 Atheroscelerosis 31; 259.

Bajusz E, ed 1966 Electrolyte and Cardiovascular Diseases: Physiology, Parthology, Therapy, vol. 2 The Williams & Wilkins Co., Baltimore.

Blahd WH et al 1963 Body potassium content in patients with muscular dystrophy - body composition part 1. Ann. N. Y. Academy of. Science. 110; 282-290.

Boegshold M Kotchen TA 1991 Importance of dietary chloride for salt sensitivity of blood pressure. Hypertension 17 (auppl) 1158-I161.

Brodsky MA et. al. 1994 Magnesium therapy in new-onset atrial fibrillation. American Journal of Cardiology 73; 1227-1229.

Brown J Bourke GJ Gearty GF Finnegan A Hill M Hefferman-Fox FC Fitzgerald DE Kennedy J Childers RW Jepsop WJE Trulson MF Latham MC Gronin S McCann MB Clancy RE Gore I & Stoudt HW 1970 Nutritional and epidemiological factors related to heart disease. World Rev. Nutr. Diet 33.

Chang HY, Hu YW, et al,2006 Effect of potassium-enriched salt on cardiovascular mortality and medical expenses of elderly men, Am J Clin Nutr, 83(6): 1289-96.

Charalampous FC 1971 Role of inositol in Na+ and K+ activated adenosine triphosphatase of KB cells. Journal of Biological Chemistry 246;455-460 and 461-465p.

Classen HG Marquardt P Spath M Schumacher KA Grabling B 1978 Experimental studies on the intestinal uptake of organic and inorganic magnesium and potassium compounds given alone or simultaneously. Arzeneim Forsch. 28 807-811.

Conway EJ 1957 Nature and significance of concentration relations of potassium and sodium ions in skelatal muscle. Phys. Rev. 37; 84.

Cope CL 1972 Adrenal Steroids and Disease, 2nd edition Lippincott Co Philadelphia.

Davis WH 1970 Does potassium deficiency hold a clue to metabolic disorders associated with liability to coronary heart disease? South African Medical Journal 44; 1297 (from the abstract).

Dumaine, R et al, 1990 Taurine Depresses I(Na) and Depolarises The

Membrane But Does Not Affect Membrane Surface Charges in Perfused Rabbit Hearts", Cardiovascular Research, 24:918-924.

FletcherGF et al 1968 Polarizing solutions in patients with myocardial infarction. American Heart Journal 75; 319.

Folis RH 1942 Myocardial necroses in rats on a potassium low diet prevented by thiamine deficiency. Bulletin Johns Hopkins Hosp.71; 235-241.

Geiss K-R, et al: 1998 Effects of Magnesium Orotate on Exercise Tolerance in Patients With Coronary Heart Disease. Cardiovascular Drugs Therapy 12:153-156.

Golf SW, et al 1998 On the Significance of Magnesium in Extreme Physical Stress. Cardiovasc Drugs Ther, 12:197-202.

Greene DA Latimer SA 1983 Impaired rat sciatic nerve sodium-potassium adenosine triphosphatase in acute streptozocin diabetes and its correction by dietary myo-inositol supplementation. Journal of Clinical Investigatio9n72; 1058-1063.

Hall JR Swaine RL 1972 Trends in the carbonated beverage industry. Critical Reviews in Food Technology, V2, issue 4; 517-536.

Harvey PW Hunsaker HA & Allen KG 1981 Dietary L-histidine induced hypercholerolemia and hypocupremia in the rat. Journal of Nutrition 111; 639.

Heianza Y et al 2011 Low serum potassium levels and risk of type 2 diabetes: the Toranomon Hospital health management Center Study 1 . Diabetologia 54; 762-766.

Howard JE & Carey RA 1949 The use of potassium in therapy. Journal Clinical Endocrinology 9; 691-713.

He FJ, Markandu ND, Coltart R, Barron J, MacGregor GA 2005. Effect of short-term supplementation of potassium chloride and potassium citrate on blood pressure in hypertensives. Hypertension.;45(4):571-574.

Ifudu O Markell MS Friedman EA 1992 Unrecognized pseudohyperkalemia as a cause of elevated potassium in patients with renal disease. American Journal of Nephrology 12; 102-104.

Kadaner Vya & Solonitsyna OP 1965 The therapeutic action of potassium chloride in patients with hypertensive and coronary disease (in Russian) in; The Pathology of the Hepato-pancreato-duodenial Zone and Disorders of Circulation.(Moscow). 66-67. From Bio Abstracts 1966 V47, p4478, Article 52531.

Khaw K-T Barrett-Connor E 1987 Dietary potassium and stroke associated mortality. 316; 235-249.

Klevay LM 1974 Interactions among dietary copper, zinc and themetabolism of cholesterol and phospholipids. P553-556. In; Hoekstra WG Suttie JW Ganther HE Mertz W eds. Trace Element Metabolism in Animals –2. University Park Press, Baltimore.

Klevay LM 1978 Hypercholesteremia in rats produced by an increase in the ratio of zinc to copper.American Journal of Clinical Nutrition 26; 1060.

Klevay LM &Viestenz KE 1981 Abnormal electrocardiogram in rats deficient in copper. American Journal of Physiol. Heart Cir. Physiol. 9; H185-H189.

Klevay LM 1987 Hypertension in rats due to copper deficiency. Nutrition Reports International 35; 999-1006.

Kohvakka A Luurila O Gordin A & Sundberg S 1989 Magnesium. Magnesium 8; 71-76.

Laborit H Huguenard P 1956 Aspects biologiques de la reanimation cardiaque et vasculaire. Applications practiques. Journal Chir. Paris 72; 681.

Laborit H et al 1958 The place of certain salts of D. L. aspartic acid in the mechanism of preservation of the activity of reaction to environment. La Presse Medicale 66; 1307.

Lau BW Klevay LM 1982 Postheparin plasma lipoprotein lipase in copper deficient rats. Journal of Nutrition 112; 928-933.

Liddle GW et al 1953 The prevention of ACTH-induced sodium retention by the use of potassium salts: a quantitative study. Journal of Clinical Investigation 32; 1197-1207.

Luderitz B 1984 Potassium deficiency and cardiac function: experimental and clinical aspects. Magnesium 3: 289-300

Lundman T & Orinius E 1965 Insulin-glucose-potassium infusion in acute myocardial infarction. Acta Med. Scand. 178; 525-528.

McDonald JT Margen S 1979 Wine vs ethanol in human nutrition. Fluid sodium and potassium balance. American journal of Clinical Nutrition 32; 817-822.

Messerli FH et al 1977 Effects of angiotensin II on steroid metabolism and hepatic blood flow in man. Circ. Res 40;204-207 Mondon CD 1968

Glucose tolerance and insulin response of potassium deficient rat and isolated liver. American Journal Physiology 215; 779-787.

Pierson RN and McCord C 1970 Total body potassium in heart disease serial changes after surgical correction. Circ. 42; 4 abstract #320.

Potter JM Blake GM Cox JR 1984 Potassium supplements and total body potassium in elderly patients. Age & Ageing 13; 238-242.

Prioreschi MD 1967 Experimental cardiac necrosis and potassium: a review. Canad. Med. Assoc. J. 96; 1221-1223.

Rackley CE et al 1979 Glucose-insulin potassium infusion. Postgrad. Med. 65; 93-99.

Romanski SA, McMahon MM. Metabolic acidosis and thiamine deficiency. Mayo Clin Proc. 1999 Mar;74(3):259-63, 1999.

Rubini ME 1961 Water excretion in potassium - deficient man. Journal of Clinical Investigation 40; 2215-2224.

Schlebusch H, et al, 1992 Bioavailability of Magnesium as Magnesium-Orotate and Magnesium- Hydroxycarbonate", Med Welt, 43; 523-8.

Schecter M Kaplinsky E Rabinowitz B 1992 The rationale of magnesium supplementation in acute myocardial infarction. A review of the literature. Arch Intern Medicine 152; 2189-2196.

Selye H, et al 1945 Experimental nephrosclerosis, prevention with ammonium chloride. Lancet 1; 301H304.

Selye H & Bajusz E 1958 Provocation and prevention of potassium deficiency by various ions. Proceedings of the Soc. Exptl. Biol. and Med. 98; 580-583.

Suter PM, Vetter W. Diuretics and vitamin B1: are diuretics a risk factor for thiamin malnutrition? Nutr. Rev. 58:319-323, 2000.

Szabo Z Arnqvist H Hokanson E Jorfeldt L Svedjehholm R 2001 Effects of high-dose glucose-insulin-potassium on myocardial metabolism after coronary surgery in patientswith type II diabetes. Clin. Sci. (London) 101; 37-43.

Thadani V Chiong MA Parker JO 1979 Effects of glucose - insulin - potassium infusion on the angina response during treadmill exercise. Cardiology 64; 333-349.

Thomson, AD Baker H Leevy CM 1971 Folate-induced malabsorption of thiamine. Gastroenterology 60, 756.

Thomson AD Frank O DeAngelis B et al 1972 Thiamine depletion induced by folate deficiency in rats. Nutrition Reports International,

Walsh CR Larson MG Liep EP Vasan RS Levy D 2002 Serum potassium and risk of cardiovascular disease. Archives of Internal Medicine 162; (9) 1002-1012.

Waxweiler RJ Wagoner JK Archer VE 1973 Mortality of Potash Workers. Journal of Occupational Medicine 15; 486-489.

Whang R Flink EB 1983 Glucose - insulin - potassium infusion in acute myocardial infarction - an overview. in; Whang R Aikawa JK eds. Potassium: its Biologic Significance. CRC Press, Boca Raton, Fl.

Whelton PK, He J, Cutler JA, Et al. 1977 Effects of oral potassium on blood pressure. Meta-analysis of randomized controlled clinical trials. JAMA. 1997;277(20):1624-1632.

White RJ 1970 Potassium supplements on the exchangeable potassium in chronic heart disease. Brit. Med. J. 3; 141-142.

CHAPTER 4: RHEUMATOID ARTHRITIS

Adamashvili I, Pressly T, Gebel H, Milford E, Wolf R, Mancini M, Sittg K, Ghali GE, Hall V, McDonald JC. 2002 Soluble HLA in saliva of patients with autoimmune rheumatic diseases. Rheumatol Int. 2002 Jun;22(2):71-6. Epub 2002 May 04.

Allander E and Buelle A 1981 Developments in epidemiological studies of rheumatoid arthritis. Scandinavian Journal of Rheumatology 10; 257-261.

Axford JS,. 2000 Glycosylation and rheumatic disease. Proceedings of the Royal Society of Medicine's 5th Jenner Symposium (Glycobiology and Medicine conference),10-11,.

Bach TF editor 1947 Arthritis and Related Conditions. FA Davis Co., Philadelphia.

Bazzichi L Ciompi ML Betti L Rossi A Melchiorre D Fiorini M Giannaccini G Lucacchini A 2002 Impaired glutathione reductase activity and levels of collagenase and elastase in synovial fluid in rheumatoid arthritis. Clin. Exp. Rheumatol. 20; 761-766.

Beeton C et al 2006: Kv1.3 channels are a therapeutic target for T cell-mediated autoimmune diseases. Proc Natl Acad Sci U S A .103(46); 17414-17419.

Best CH & Taylor NB 1960 The Physiological Basis of Medical Practice, 5th ed. Williams & Wilkins Co. Baltimore.

Boegshold M Kotchen TA 1991 Importance of dietary chloride for salt sensitivity of blood pressure. Hypertension 17 (auppl) 1158-I161.

Casatta L Ferraccioli GF & Bartoli E 1997 Hypokalaemic alkalosis, acquired Gitelman's and Barter's syndrome in chronic sialoadenitis. British Journal of Rheumatology 36; 1125-1128.

Chen I 1995 The diagnostic significance of rheumatoid factors in patients with early rheumatoid arthritis. Chung Hua Nei Ko Tsq Chih 34 (7); 449-451 (from abstract).

Cockel R, Kendall MJ, Becker JF, Hawkins CF 1971 Serum biochemical values in rheumatoid disease. Ann Rheum Dis; 30(2):166-70.

Crain DC 1959 Help for Ten Million, 1st edition. JP Lippicott Co, NY.

Das UN 2000 Newer uses of glucose-insulin-potassium regime. Med Sci. Monit. 6; 1053-1055.

DeCoti-Marsh C 1994 Rheumatism and Arthritis: the Conquest. Amberwood Publishers, lmt.Rochester, Kent UK tel. 01634 290115.

Deessein PH Joffe BL Stanwic AE Moomal Z 2001 Hyposecretion of the adrenal androgen dehydroepiandrosterone sulfate and its relation to chemical variables in inflammatory arthritis. Arthritis Research 3; 183-188.

Dong CH & Banks J 1975 New Hope for the Arthritic. Ballantine Books, NY.

Dorup I Skajaa K Thybo NK 1994 Oral magnesium supplementation to patients receiving diuretics-normalization of magnesium, potassium and sodium pumps in the skeletal muscles. Ugeskr Laeger 156; 4007-4013 (article in Danish.

Durlach J Colery P 1984 Magnesium and potassium in diabetes and carbohydrate metabolism. Review of the present status and recent results. Magnesium 3; 315 323.

Eppinger H 1939 Einiges uber diatische therapie. Ztschr. F. Arzneimittelforschung 672-678 & 709-714.

Fujita A Hashimoto Y Nakahara K Tanaka T Okuda T & Koda M 1999 Effects of a low calorie vegan diet on disease activity and general conditions in patients with rheumatoid arthritis. Rinsho Byori 47; 554-560.

Garay RP Dagher G Pernollet MG Dovynck MA Meyer P 1980 Inherited defect in a Na+, K-co-transport system in erythrocytes from essential hypertensive patients. Nature 284; 281-283.

Halpern ML Goldstein MB 1999 Fluid, Electrolyte, and Acid-base Physiology. WB Saunders, Philadelphia.

Helmick CG Lawrence RC Pollard RA Lloyd E Heyse S 1995 Arthritis and other rheumatic conditions: who is affected now and who will be affected later? Arthritis Care and Research. 3.

Hofstrom I et al 2001 A vegan diet free of gluten improves the signs and symptoms of rheumatoid arthritis: the effects on arthritis correlate with a reduction in antibodies to food antigens. Rheumatology 40; 1175-1179.

Holbrook AA 1944 The raw food diet: A therapeutic agent. Ann. Int. Med. 20; 512.

Imrich R Rovensky J Malis F Zlnay M KillingerZ Kvetnansky R Huckova M Vigas M Macho L Koska J 2005 Low levels of dehydroepiandrosterone sulphate in plasma, and reduced sympathoadrenal response to hypoglycaemia in premenopausal women with rheumatoid arthritis. Annals of the Rheumatic Diseases 64: 202-206.

Jager W de, Esther P A H Hoppenreijs Wulffraat NM, Wedderburn LR Kuis W Prakken BJ 2007 Blood and synovial fluid cytokine signatures in patients with juvenile idiopathic arthritis: a cross-sectional study, Annals of the Rheumatic Diseases 66: 589-598.

Jarvis DC 1960 Arthritis and Folk Medicine. Pan Books Limited, London.

Kellgren JH 1966 Epidemiology of RA. Arthritis and Rheumatism 9; 658-674.

Khetagurova ZV 1982 Function of the hypothalamic-hypophyseal-adrenal system in patients with rheumatoid arthritis. Terapevticheskii Archiv 54; 92-95. (Russian).

Kjeldsen-kragh 1999 Rheumatoid arthritis treated with vegetarian diets. American Journal of Clinical Nutrition, 70, No. 3, 594S-600S.

Kremer JM Bigouette J 1996 Nutrient intake of patients with rheumatoid arthritis is deficient in pyridoxine, zinc, copper, and magnesium. J.of Rheumatology 23; 990-994.

La Vecchia C, Decarli A, Pagano R 1998 Vegetable consumption and risk of chronic disease Epidemiology 9(2):208-210.

LaCelle PL et al 1964 An investigation of total body potassium in patients with rheumatoid arthritis. Proceedings Ann. Meeting of the Rheumatism Association, Arthritis & Rheumatism 7; 321.

LaMont Havers RW 1963 Nutrition and the rheumatic diseases, part II, Collagen diseases. Borden's Review of Nutrition Research 24; 15-27.

Linos A et al. 1999 Dietary factors in relation to rheumatoid arthritis: a role for olive oil and cooked vegetables? American Journal of Clinical Nutrition 70: 1077-82.

Luft FC Zemel MB Sowers JA Fineberg NS Weinberger MH 1990 Sodium bicarbonate and sodium chloride: effects on blood pressure and electrolyte homeostasis in normal and hypertensive man. Journal of Hypertension 8; 663-670.

Masoom-Yasinzai M 1996 Altered fatty acid, cholesterol. and Na/K ATPase activity in erythrocyte membrane of rheumatoid arthritis patients. Zeitschrift fur Naturforschung, section C, Bioscience 51; 401-403 (from the abstract).

Morgan SL Anderson AM Hood SM Mathews PA Lee JY Alarcon GS 1997 Nutrient intake patterns, body mass index, and vitamin levels in patients with rheumatoid arthritis. Arthritis Care Research 10; 9-17. (from abstract).

Narins RG 1994 Clinical Disorders of Fluid and Electrolyte Metabolism. McGraw Hill, inc. New York City.

NHANES-III, Catalog #77560, U.S. Department of Health and Human Services (DHHS). National Center for Health Statistics. Third National Health and Nutrition Examination Survey, 1988-1994, NHANES III Laboratory Data File (CD-ROM). Public Use Data File Documentation Number 76200. Hyattsville, MD.: Centers for Disease Control and Prevention, 1996. Available from; National Technical Information Service (NTIS), Springfield, VA. Acrobat. PDF format; includes access software: Adobe Systems, Inc. Acrobat Reader 2.1.

Osol A Farrar GE United States Dispensatory, 25th edition, Part I. JP Lippencott & Co., Philadelphia.

Phelps AE Your Arthritis: What You Can Do About It. Wm. Morrow & Co., NY.

Rasch EK Hirsch R Paulose-Ram R Hochberg MC.2003 Prevalence of rheumatoid arthritis in persons 60 years of age and older in the United States: effect of different methods of case classification. Arthritis Rheum. 2003 Apr;48(4):917-26.

Rastmanesh R 2008 A pilot study of potassium supplementation in treatment of hypokalemic patients with rheumatoid arthritis: a randomized, double-blinded, placebo controlled trial. The Journal of Pain 9; 722-731.

Riley JP 1961 Composition of mineral water from the hot spring at Bath. Journal of Applied Chemistry 11; 190-192.

Roberts-Thomson RA Roberts-Thomson PJ. 1999 Rheumatic disease and the Australian aborigine. Ann Rheum Dis. May 58: 266-70. Rodman GP editor. Primer on the Rheumatic Diseases, 7th edition. The Arthritis Foundation, NY.

Ropes MW et al 1958 Revision of diagnostic criteria for rheumatoid arthritis. Bull. Rheum. Dis. 9; 175.

Rubini ME 1961 Water excretion in potassium - deficient man. Journal of Clinical Investigation 40; 2215-2224.

Sambrook PN Ansell BM Foster S Gumpel JM Hesp R Reeve J Zanelli JM 1985 Bone turnover in early rheumatoid arthritis. 1. Biochemical and kinetic indexes.Ann Rheum Dis. 44(9):575-579.

Sobel D Klein AC Arthritis What Works, St. Martin's Press, 175 Fifth Ave. NY.

Sari I Astorga G Carvagal P Gatica H 1993 Clinical usefulness of rheumatoid factor in synovial fluid, reevaluation. Rev. Med. Chil 121: 1374-1378 (from abstract).

Schubert J 1966 Chelation in medicine. Scientific American 214; 40.

Shin S, Furin J, Alcántara F, Hyson A, Joseph K, Sánchez E, Rich M. 2004 Hypokalemia among patients receiving treatment for multidrug-resistant tuberculosis. Chest. Mar;125(3): 974-980.

Siamopoulou A Mavridis AK Vasakos AK Benecos P Tzioufas AG Andonopoulos AP 1989 Sialochemistry in juvenile chronic arthritis. British Journal of Rheumatology 28; 383-385 (from the abstract).

Silman AJ Ollier W Holligan S Birrell F Adebajo A Asuzu MC Thomson W Pepper L 1993 Absence of rheumatoid arthritis in a rural Nigerian population. Journal of Rheumatology. 20(4): 618-622.

Straub et al 2002 Inadequately low serum levels of steroid hormones in relation to interleukin-6 and tumor necrosis factor in untreated patients with early rheumatoid arthritis and reactive arthritis. Arthritis Rheum. 46; 654-662.

Strukov A 1964 General morphology of collagen diseases. Journal of Pathology 78; 409-420.

Stone J Doube A Dudson D Wallace J 1997 Inadequate calcium. folic acid. vitamin E zinc, and selenium intake in rheumatoid arthritis patients: results of a dietary survey. Seminars in Arthritis and Rheum. 27; 180-185.

Sukenik S Neumann L Buskila D Kleiner-Baumgarten A Zimlichman S Horowitz J 1990 Dead sea bath salts or the treatment of rheumatoid arthritis. Clinical Exp. Rheumatology 8; 353-357 (from the abstract).

Syrjanen S Lappalainen R Markkanen H 1986 Salivary and serum levels of electrolytes and immunomarkers in edentulous healthy subjects and in those with rheumatoid arthritis. Clinical Rheumatology 5; 49-55.

Testa I Rabini RA Corvetta A Danieli G 1987 Decreased sodium, potassium ATPase activity in erythrocyte membrane from rheumatoid arthritis patients. Scandinavian Journal of Rheumatology 16; 301-305.

Trujillo E Alvarez de la Rosa D Mobasheri A Gonzolez T Canessa CM Martin-Vasallo P 1999 Sodium transport systems in human chondrocytes II. Expression of ENaC, Na+/K+/2Cl cotransporter Na+/H+ exchangers in healthy and arthritic chondrocytes. Histol. Histopathol. 14; 1023-1031 (from the abstract).

Trang LE Furst P Odeback AC Lovgren O 1985 Plasma amino acids in rheumatoid arthritis. Scandinavian Rheumatology 14; 393-402.

Veinpalu E Trink RF Veinpalu LE Pyder KhA 1992 The therapeutic action of the low water bulk of sea mud. Vopr.Kurortol. Fizioter Lech Fiz. Kult. Sep.-Dec.;(5-6); 54-57.

Waller 1971 Present status of rheumatoid factor. Crit. Rev. Clin. Lab . Sci 2; 173-210.

Winegrad AT Reynold AE 1958 Effect of insulin on the metabolism of glucose, pyruvate, and acetate. Journal of Biological. Chemistry 233; 267.

CHAPTER 5; GOUT

Batuman V Maesaka JK Landy E Haddad B Wedeen P Tepper E 1981 The role of lead in gout nephropathy. New England Journal of Medicine 304; 520-3.

Blau LW.1950 Cherry diet control for gout and arthritis. Tex Rep Biol Med 8:309-11.

Colton RS Ward LE 1966 Uric acid, gout, and the kidney. Medical Clinics of North America 50, o. 4; 1031-1042.

Gonzalez JJ et al 1979 Renin aldosterone system and potassium levels in chronic lead intoxication. South Med. Journal 72; 433-436.

Greenly L 2003 An overview of antihypertensive medications and assessing blood pressure using the latest guidelines. Journal of Chiropractic Medicine 2; 117 123.

Jacob RA, Spinozzi GM, Simon VA, Kelley DS, Prior RL, Hess-Pierce B, Kader AA. 2003 Consumption of cherries lowers plasma urate in healthy women. J Nutr. 133(6); 1826-1829.

Kiohara C, et al 1999 Inverse association between coffee drinking and serum uric acid concentration in middle - aged Japanese males. British Medical Journal 82; 125-130.

Lin JL Yu CC Lin-Tan DT Ho HH 2001 Lead chelation therapy and urate excretion in patients with chronic renal diseases and gout. Kidney Int. 60(1):266-71.

Lin JL, Tan DT, Ho HH, Yu CC 2002 Environmental lead exposure and urate excretion in the general population. Am J Med. 113(7):563-8.

Naohiko Anzai, Atsushi Enomoto and Hitoshi Endou 2005 Renal Urate Handling: Clinical Relevance of Recent Advances. Current Rheumatology Reports 7; 227-234.

Rodman JS 2002 Intermittant versus continuous alkaline therapy for uric acid stones and uretal stones of uncertain composition. Urology 60; 378-382.

Shekarriz B, Stoller ML 2002 Uric acid nephrolithiasis: current concepts and controversies. J Urol. 2002 Oct;168 (4 Pt 1): 1307-14.

Turner RA Counts GB Treadway WJ Holt DA Agudelo CA 1981 Rheumatoid factor and monosodium urate crystal-neutrophil interactions in gouty inflammation. Inflammation 5; 353-361.

Wright, LF; Saylor, RP; Ceere, FA (1984) Occult lead intoxication in patients with gout and kidney disease. Journal of Rheumatology. 11, no. 4; 517-520.

CHAPTER 6: DIABETES

Ahuja KDK Lennon DP Greenwood MR Buckenham AJ 2006 Effects of chili consumption on postprandial glucose, insulin, and energy metabolism. American Journal of Clinical Nutrition 84; 63-69.

Allard J, Lennon DP, Greenwood MR, Buckenham AJ, Hawthorne JN. 1993 Reduced sodium pump activity in inositol-deficient HL-60 cells: no evidence of control by protein kinase C. Biochim Biophys Acta. Dec 16;1220(1): 66-68.

Andersen HU, et al. 1994 Nicotinamide prevents interleukin-1 effects on accumulated insulin release and nitric oxide production in rat islets of langerhans. Diabetes 43, 770-777.

Anderson RA, et al. Dietary chromium intake: freely chosen diets, institutional diets, and individual foods. Biol Trace Elem Res 1992;32:117-21.

Anderson RA, et al. 1997a Elevated intakes of supplemental chromium improve glucose and insulin variables with type 2 diabetes. Diabetes;46:1786-91.

Anderson RA, et al. 1997b Lack of toxicity of chromium chloride and chromium picolinate. J Am Coll Nutr;16:273-279.

Atkins RC 2003 New Diet Revolution, Vermilion .

Babaei-Jadidi R Karachalias N Ahmed N, Battah S, Thornalley PJ 2003 Prevention of Incipient Diabetic Nephropathy by High-Dose Thiamine and Benfotiamine. Diabetes 52; 2110-2120.

Balzer J et al 2008 Awadallah R, El-Dessoukey EA, Doss H, Khalifa K, el-Hawary Z 1978 Blood-reduced glutathione, serum ceruloplasmin and mineral changes in juvenile diabetes. Z Ernahrungswiss 17(2):79-83.

Balzer J et al 2008 Sustained Benefits in Vascular Function Through Flavanol-Containing Cocoa in Medicated Diabetic Patients. Journal of American College of Cardiology. 51; 2141-2149.

Barbagallo M Dominguez LJ Galioto A Ferlisi A Cani C Malfa L Pineo A Busardo' A Paolisso G 2003 Role of magnesium in insulin action, diabetes and cardio-metabolic syndrome X. Mol Aspects Med. 2003 ;24(1-3): 39-52.

Barger AC Berlin RD Tulenko JF 1958. Infusion of aldosterone, 9 alpha fluorohydrocortisone, and antidiuretic hormone into the renal artery of normal and adrenalectomized unaesthetized dogs: effect on electrolyte and water excretion. Endocrinology 62; 804,

Bartlett GR MacKay EM 1949 Insulin stimulation of glycogen formation in rat abdominal muscle. Proc. Soc. Exp. Biol. Med. 71; 493-495.

Bian J Cui J McDonald TV 2001 Herg K+ channel is regulated y changes in phosphatidyl inositol 4,5-bisphosphate. Circulation Research. 89(12): 1168-76.

Bihari B 1995 Efficacy of low dose Naltrexone as an immune stabilizing agent for treatment of HIV/AIDS [letter] AIDS Patient Care 9; 3.

Blanchard, JF Armenian HK Friesen PP 2000 Risk Factors for Abdominal Aortic Aneurysm: Results of a Case-Control Study. American Journal of Epidemiology 151(6); 575-583.

Boegshold M Kotchen TA 1991 Importance of dietary chloride for salt sensitivity of blood pressure. Hypertension 17 (suppl) I 158-I161.

Chan JM, Stampfer MJ, Ma J, Gann PH, Gaziano JM, Giovannucci EL. 2001 Dairy products, calcium, and prostate cancer risk in the Physicians' Health Study. Am J Clin Nutr 74(4):549-54.

Charansonney OL Jean-Pierre Després J-P 2010 Disease prevention—should we target obesity or sedentary lifestyle? Nature Reviews Cardiology 7, 468-472.

Chattergee R et al 2010 Serum and dietary potassium and risk of incident type 2 diabetes mellitus. Arch. Intern. Med.170; 1745-1751.

Choi SW Benzie IF Lam CS Chat SW Lam J Yiu CH Kwan JJ Tang YH Yeung GS Yeung VT Woo GC Hannigan BM Strain JJ 2005 Inter-relationships between DNA damage, ascorbic acid and glycaemic control in Type 2 diabetes mellitus. Diabet. Med. (10) 1347-1353.

Choi HK, Walter C. Willett, Meir J. Stampfer, Eric Rimm, Frank B. Hu, 2005 Dairy Consumption and Risk of Type 2 Diabetes Mellitus in Men. Arch Intern Med. 2005; 165: 997-1003.

Cohen AM Teitelbaum A Miller E Ben-tor V Hirt R Fields M 1982 Effect of copper on carbohydrate metabolism in rats. Isr. J. Med. Sci. 18; 840-844.

Colditz GA Manson JE Stampfer MJ Rosner B Willett WC Speizer FE 1992 Diet and risk of clinical diabetes in women. American Journal of Clinical Nutrition 55; 1018-1023.

Craft NE & Failla 1983 Zinc, iron, and copper absorption in the streptozotocin-diabetic rat. American Journal of Physiology 244; E 122-128.

Das UN 2000 Newer uses of glucose-insulin-potassium regimen. Med. Sci. Monit. 6(6); 1053-1055.

Debons AF Krimsky I Fromm A 1970 A direct action of insulin on the hypothalamic satiety center. American Journal of Physiology 219; 938-?.

Dhatariya K Bigelow ML Nair KS 2005 Effect of dehydrocepiandrosterone replacement on insulin sensitivity and lipids in hypoadrenal women. Diabetes 54; 765-769.

Di Leo MAS . Santini SA. Cercone S Lepore D Gentiloni Silveri N Caputo S. Greco AV Giardina B. Franconi F Ghirlanda G 2000 Chronic taurine supplementation ameliorates oxidative stress and $Na^+K^+ATPase$ impairment in the retina of diabetic rats. Amino Acids 23; 401-406.

Di Leo MA, Ghirlanda G, Gentiloni Silveri N, Giardina B, Franconi F, Santini SA. 2003 Potential therapeutic effect of antioxidants in experimental diabetic retina: a comparison between chronic taurine and vitamin E plus selenium supplementations. Free Radical Res. 2003 Mar;37(3):323-30.

Durlach J Colery P 1984 Magnesium and potassium in diabetes and carbohydrate metabolism. Review of the present status and recent results. Magnesium 3; 315 323.

Elliott SS L Keim N Stern JS Teff K Havel PJ 2002 Fructose, weight gain, and the insulin resistance syndrome American Journal of Clinical Nutrition, 76; 911-922.

Elliott RB Pilcher CC Fergusson DM Stewart AW 1996 A population based strategy to prevent insulin-dependent diabetes using nicotinamide. J Pediatr Endocrinol Metab. ;9(5):501-9.

Engelen W et al 2000 Effects of long-term supplementation with moderate pharmacologic doses of vitamin E are saturable and reversible in patients with type 1 diabetes. American Journal of Clinical Nutrition 72; 1142-1149.

Fell BF 1982 Pancreatic atrophy in copper-deficient rats: histochemical and ultrastructural evidence of a selective effect on acinar cells. Histochem. Journal 14; 665-80.

Flatman JA Clausen T 1979 Combined effects of adrenaline and insulin on active electrogenic Na^+-K^+ transport in rat soleus muscle. Nature 281; 580-581.

Folis RH 1942 Myocardial necroses in rats on a potassium low diet prevented by thiamine deficiency. Bulletin Johns Hopkins Hosp.71; 235-241.

Franconi F Loizzo A Ghirlanda G Sighieri G 2006 Taurine supplementation and diabetes mellius. Curr. Opin. Clinical Nutr. Metab. Care 9 (1); 32-36.

Fung TT Hi FB Pereira MA Liu S Stampfer MJ Colditz GA, et al 2002 Whole grain intake and the risk of type 2 diabetes; A prospective study in man. American Journal of Clinical Nutrition 76 (3); 535-540.

Fujita T Ando K Nod H Ito Y Sato Y 1987 Effects of increased adrenomedullary activity and taurine in young patients with borderline hypertension. Circulation 75; 525-532.

Gale EA 1996 Theory and practice of nicotinamide trials in pre-type 1 diabetes. J. Pediatr. Endocrinol. Metab. 8(3); 375-379.

Gardner LI 1953 Experimental potassium depletion. Journal Lancet 73; 190.

Garrow J Garrow R 2003 Human Nutrition & Dietetics, 10th Edition, Churchill Livingstone.

Gassman CA Failla ML Osborne SP Alexander AR 1983 Copper accumulation in the soluble and particulate fractions of renal cortex in the streptozotocin-diabetic rat. Biological Trace Element Research 5; 475-487.

Gibbs WW 2005 Obesity: An overblown epidemic. Scientific American 292; 70-77.

Gould SE, ed 1968 Pathology of the Heart and Blood Vessels - 3rd ed. Charles C. Thomas, Springfield, Ill 508.

Haskins K, et al 2003 Immunology of diabetes II: Pathogenesis from mouse o man. Ann. N.Y. Academy of Sciences Volume 1005 published November 2003 Ann. N.Y. Acad. Sci. 1005: 43. doi: 10.1196/annals.1288.006.

Havas M 2006 Electromagnetic hypersensitivity: biological effects of dirty electricity with emphasis on diabetes and multiple sclerosis. Electromagn Biol Med. ;25(4):259-68.

Helderman JH et al 1983 Prevention of the glucose intolerance of thiazide diuretics by maintenance of body potassium. Diabetes 32; 106-111.

Hoffmaan A Zif E 1997 Pharmacokinetic considerations of new insulin formulations and routes of administration. Cin. Pharmacokinet. 33; 285-301.

Hollis BW 2005 Circulating 25-Hydroxyvitamin D Levels Indicative of Vitamin D Sufficiency: Implications for Establishing a New Effective Dietary Intake Recommendation for Vitamin D[1] Journal of Nutrition 135; 317-322.

Houck JC Sharma VK Patel YM Gladner JA. 1968.Induction of collagenolytic & proteolytic activities by anti-inflammatory drugs in the skin and fibroblasts. Biochem. Pharmacology. 17; 2081,

Houstis N 2006 Reactive oxygen species have a causal role in multiple forms of insulin resistance. Nature 440; 944.

Hypponen E Laara E Reunanen A Jarvelio ME Virtamen SM 2001 Intake of vitamin D and risk of type 1 diabetes: a birth-cohort study. Lancet 358 (9292); 1500-1503.

Hyppönen E Läärä E Reunanen A Järvelin MR Virtanen SM 2001 Intake of vitamin D and risk of type 1 diabetes: a birth-cohort study. Lancet. 2001 358(9292):1500-3.

Jayaprakasam B Vareed SK Olson LK Nair MG 2005 Insulin Secretion by Bioactive Anthocyanins and Anthocyanidins Present in Fruits. Journal of Agric. Food Chem., 53 (1), 28 –31.

Jain HK Lim G 2001 Pyridoxine and pyridoxamine inhibits superoxide radicals and prevents lipid peroxidation, protein glycosylation, and (Na$^+$ + K$^+$)-ATPase activity reduction in high glucose-treated human erythrocytes. Free Radical Biology and Medicine 30; 232-237.

JNCI 2002 More Than Spice: Capsaicin in Hot Chili Peppers Makes Tumor Cells Commit Suicide. Journal of the National Cancer Institute 94; 1263-1265.

Jovanovic-Peterson L, Peterson CM. 1996 Vitamin and mineral deficiencies which may predispose to glucose intolerance of pregnancy. J Am Coll Nutr. Feb;15(1):14-20.

Kao WHL et al 1999 Serum and dietary magnesium and the risk for type 2 diabetes mellitus. Archives of Internal Medicine 159.

Khan A 2003 Cinnamon Improves Glucose and Lipids of People With Type 2 Diabetes. Diabetes Care 26; 3215 – 3218.

Kimball SM Ursell MR O'Connor P Vieth R 2007 Safety of vitamin D3 in adults with multiple sclerosis. American Journal of Clinical Nutrition. 86; 645-651.

Knochel JP 1977 Role of glucoregulatory hormones in potassium homeostasis. Kidney International 11; 443, 1977.

Knochel JP 1984 Diuretic induced hypokalemia. Am J Med.;77(5A):18-27.

Kolb H Burkhart V 1999 Nicotinamide in type 1 diabetes. Mechanism of action revisited. Diabetes Care Suppl. 2; B16-20.

LaCelle PL et al 1964. An investigation of whole body potassium in patients with rheumatoid arthritis. Proceedings Annual Meeting of the American Rheumatism Association. Arthritis & Rheumatism 7;327, - or New England Journal of Medicine 311; 1214, 1984.

Laires MJ Monteiro CP Bicho M 2004 Role of cellular magnesium in health human disease. Frontiers in Bioscience 9, 262-276.

Lamer J 2002 D-chiro-inositol—its functional role in insulin action and its deficit in insulin resistance. Int J Exp Diabetes Res. 2002; 3(1): 47-60.

Lans HS et al 1952 The relation of serum potassium to erythrocyte potassium in normal subjects and patients with potassium deficiency. American Journal Med. Sci. 223; 65-74.

Laitinen K, Poussa T, Isolauri E 2009 Probiotics and dietary counselling contribute to glucose regulation during and after pregnancy: a randomised controlled trial. Br J Nutr. 101:1679-1687.

Lazarow A., Liambies L., and Tausch AJ, 1950 Protection against diabetes with nicotinamide. J. Lab. Clin. Med. 36, 249-258.

Lee D H et al 2004 Does supplemental vitamin C increase cardiovascular disease risk in women with diabetes? American journal of 80; 1194-1200.

Lee D Lee I Jin S Steffes M Jacobs DR Jr. 2007 Association Between Serum Concentrations of Persistent Organic Pollutants and Insulin Resistance Among Nondiabetic Adults. Diabetes Care 30; 622-628.

Li W Tian Y Feng H Tu B 1998 Effects of taurine and extraction of cristata L on serum Zn, Cu and Ca in rats. Wei Sheng Yan Jiu (Journal of Hygiene Research) 30, 27(5) 341-243. (article in Chinese).

Lungberg M Korpela R Ilonen J Ludvigsson J Vaarala O 2006 Probiotics for the Prevention of Beta Cell Autoimmunity in Children at Genetic Risk of Type 1 Diabetes. the PRODIA Study. Ann N Y Acad Sci. Oct;1079: 360-4.

Luoto R, Laitinen K, Nermes M, Isolauri E. 2010 Impact of maternal probiotic-supplemented dietary counselling on pregnancy outcome and prenatal and postnatal growth: a double-blind, placebo-controlled study. Br J Nutr. 2010 Jun;103(12):1792-9. .

Lutsey PL Steffen LM Stevens J 2008 Dietary intake and the development of the metabolic syndrome. Circulation 117; 754-761.

Mandrup PT, et al., 1993 Nicotinamide in the prevention of insulin dependent diabetes mellitus. Diabetes Metabol Rev., 9, 295-309.

Marcus DF et al 1968 A comparative study of various hyperglycemic agents in potassium deficient rats. Proceedings of the Society Experimental Biol. Med. 127; 533-538.

Masterjohn C 2007 vitamin D toxicity redefined: vitamin K and the molecular mechanism. Medical Hypotheses 68; 1026-1034.

McCarty 2004 Should we restrict chloride rather than sodium? Medical Hypotheses 63; 138-148.

McCarty MF 2005 Chromium picolinate may favorably influence the vascular risk associated with smoking by combating cortisol-induced insulin resistance. Medical Hypotheses 64; 1220-1224.

McCarty MF 2006 Rationale for a novel neutraceutical complex K-water: potassium taurine bicarbonate (PTB) Medical Hypotheses 67; 65-70.

McCarty MF 2007 Exenatide and biotin in conjunction with a protein sparing fast for normalization of beta cell function in type 2 diabetes. Medical Hypotheses 69; 928-932.

Mineno T 1969 Effect of some vitamins and other substances on K metabolism in the myocardia of vitamin deficient rats - Experimetal investigation. J. Nagoya Med. Assoc. 92; 80-95.

Mondon CD 1968 Glucose tolerance and insulin response of potassium deficient rat and isolated liver. American Journal Physiology 215; 779-787.

Moore RD 1986 Role of intracellular pH in insulin action. P?-290. In; Aronson PS Boron WF eds. Na-H Exchange, Intracellular pH, and Cell Function. Academic Press, Orlando.

Moore RD Fidelman ML Hanson JC Otis JN 1991 Role of intracellular pH in insulin action. Kroc. Found Ser. 15; 385-416.

Nadler JL Buchanen T Natarjan R Antonipillai Bergman R Rude R 1993 Magnesium deficiency produces insulin resistance and increased thromboxane synthesis. Hypertension 21; 1024-1029.

Nagabhushan M Bhide SV 1985 Mutagenicity of chili extract and capsaicin in short-term tests. Environ. Mutagen. 7; 881-888.

National Research Council. Recommended dietary allowances. 10th ed. Washington (DC): National Academy Press; 1989. p 241-2.

Norbioto G Bevilaqua M Meroni R Raggi U Dagani R Scorza DE Frigeni G Vago T 1988 Effects of potassium supplementation on insulin binding and insulin action in human obesity: protein-modified fast and refeeding. Life Sci. 42; 1323-30.

Odetti PCP et al 2003 Comparative Trial of N-Acetyl-Cysteine, Taurine, and Oxerutin on Skin and Kidney Damage in Long-Term Experimental Diabetes. Diabetes 52: 499-505.

Ozcan U et al 2006 Chemical chaperones reduce ER stress and restore glucose homeostasis in a mouse model of type 2 diabetes. Science 213; 1137-1140

Patrizio Odetti P Carlo Pesce Traverso N et al 2003 Comparative Trial of N-Acetyl-Cysteine, Taurine, and Oxerutin on Skin and Kidney Damage in Long-Term Experimental Diabetes Diabetes 52:499-505

Perry L et al 2007 Starch fossils and domestication and dispersal of Chili peppers (Capsicum spp. L.) in the Americas. Science 315;986

Pfeiffer CC Iliev V 1972 A study of zinc deficiency and copper excess in the schizophrenias. Int. Rev. Neurobiol. Supplement 1; 141-165.

Pitchford P 2002 Healing with whole foods", North Atlantic Books.

Polydefkis M 2004 The time course of epidermal nerve fibre regeneration: studies in normal controls and in people with diabetes, with and without neuropathy. Brain 127; 1606-1615.

Reid JM et al 1971 Nutrient intake of Pima Indian women: relationships to diabetes mellitus and gallbladder disease. American Journa of Clinical Nutrition 24; 1281-1289.

Reddi A DeAngelis B Frank O Lasker N Baker H 1988 Biotin supplementation improves glucose and insulin tolerances in genetically diabetic KK mice. Life Sci. 42(13); 1323-1330.

Reid JM Fullmer SD Karen D Pettigrew KD Burch TA Bennett PH Miller M Whedon GD Nutrient intake of Pima Indian women: relationships to diabetes mellitus and gallbladder disease American Journal of Clinical Nutrition, Vol 24, 1281-1289.

Rigacci S et al 2010 Oleuropein aglycon prevents cytotoxic amyloid aggregation of human amylin. Journal of Nutritional Biochemistry, 21; 726-735.

Ritchie G, Kerstan D, Dai LJ, Kang HS, Canaff L, Hendy GN, Quamme GA 2001 1,25(OH)(2)D(3) stimulates Mg2+ uptake into MDCT cells: modulation by extracellular Ca2+ and Mg2+. Am J Physiol Renal Physiol. 2001 May;280(5):F868-78.

Rowe JW et al 1980 Effect of experimental potassium deficiency on glucose and insulin metabolism. Metabolism 29; 448-502.

Ruus P et al 1999 Oral administration of rac-☒-lipoic acid modulates insulin sensitivity in patients with type-2 diabetes mellitus: a placebo-controlled pilot trial. Free Radical Biology and Medicine 27; 309-314.

Sankar D, Rao MR, et al, 2006 A pilot study of open label sesame oil in hypertensive diabetics, J Med Food, 9(3): 408-12.

Sima AAF et al 2005 Acetyl-l-Carnitine improves pain, nerve regeneration, and vibratory perception in Patients With Chronic Diabetic Neuropathy: An analysis of two randomized placebo-controlled trials. Diabetes Care 28: 89-94.

Sitasawad S, et al 2001 Beneficial effect of supplementation with copper sulfate on STZ diabetic mice (IDDM). Diabetes Res Clin Pract May;52(2):77-84.

Smith PA Sunter JP Case RM 1982 Progressive Atrophy of Pancreatic Acinar Tissue in Rats Fed a Copper-Deficient Diet Supplemented with D-Penicillamine or Triethylene Tetramine: Morphological and Physiological Studies. Digestion 23; 16-30.

Song MK,et al. 2003 Antidiabetic actions of arachidonic acid and zinc in genetically diabetic Goto-Kakizaki rats. Metabolism. 2003 52(1): 7-12.

Soffritti P et al 2006 First Experimental Demonstration of the Multipotential Carcinogenic Effects of Aspartame Administered in the Feed to Sprague-Dawley Rats. Environmental Health Perspectives 114(3)

Spergel et al 1967 Potassium on the impaired glucose tolerance in chronic uremia metabolism. Metabol. Clin. Ex. 16; 581-585.

Suresh Y , Das UN 2003 Long-chain polyunsaturated fatty acids and chemically induced diabetes mellitus. Effect of omega-3 fatty acids. Nutrition, 19(3): 213-28.

Suth Y-J 2002 More Than Spice: Capsaicin in Hot Chili Peppers Makes Tumor Cells Commit Suicide. Journal of the National Cancer Institute, Vol. 94, No. 17, 1263-1265.

Tavera-Mendoza LE White JH 2007 Cell defenses and the sunshine vitamin. Scientific American 297; 62-72.

Vieth R 1999 Vitamin D supplementation, 25-hydroxyvitamin D concentrations and safety. American Journal of Clinical Nutrition 69; 842-856.

Thornalley P. et al. (2007) High prevalence of low plasma thiamine concentration in diabetes linked to a marker of vascular disease. Diabetologia 50:2164–2170.

Trachtman HS et al 1995 Taurine ameliorates chronic streptozocin-induced diabetic nephropathy in rats. Am J Physiol Renal Physiol 269: F429-F438.

Villereal DTHollaszy JO 2004 Effect of DHEA on abdominal fat and insulin action in elderly women and men: a randomized controlled trial. JAMA 292; 2243-2248.

Vague PH, et al., 1987 Nicotinamide may extend remission phase in insulin dependent diabetes. Lancet I, 619,

Visalli N, et al 1999 A multi-centre randomized trial of two different doses of nicotinamide in patients with recent-onset type 1 diabetes (the IMDIAB VI). Diabetes Metab. Res. Rev. 15 (3); 181-185.

Von Harrath M 2009 A virus-gene collaboration. Nature 459; 518.

Wallace DC. 1997.Mitochondrial DNA in aging and disease. Scientific American 277; 40-59,

Wang W, Soltero L, Zhang P, Huang XR, Lan HY, Adrogue HJ. Renal inflammation is modulated by potassium in chronic kidney disease: possible role of Smad7. Am J Physiol Renal Physiol 2007.

Waugh A Grant A 1991/2003 Anatomy and Physiology in Health and Illness, 9th edition, Ross and Wilson.

Weber CE 2008 Does capsaicin in chili cause diabetes? Medical Hypotheses 71; 323-324.

Whang R Sims G 2000 Magnesium and potassium supplementation in the prevention of diabetic vascular disease. Medical Hypotheses 55; 263-265.

Yadav H Jain S Sinha PR 2007 Antidiabetic effect of probiotic dahi containing Lactobacillus acidophilus and Lactobacillus casei in high fructose fed rats. Nutrition; 23; :62-68.

Yadav H Jain S Sinha PR 2008 Oral administration of dahi containing probiotic Lactobacillus acidophilus and Lactobacillus casei delayed the progression of streptozotocin-induced diabetes in rats. J Dairy Res;75: 189-195.

Yared Z Chiasson JL 2003 Ketoacidosis and the hyperosmolar hyperglycemic state in adult diabetic patients. Diagnosis and treatment. Minerva Med. 2003 Dec;94(6):409-18.

Zhao HX et al 2001 Drinking water composition and childhood-onset Type 1 diabetes mellitus in Devon and Cornwall, England. Diabetic Med 18(9); 709-717.

Zheng F et al 2002 Prevention of nephropathy in mice by a diet low in glycoxidation products. Diabetes Metab. Res Rev. 18; 224-237.

Zhou Q, et al 2008 In vivo reprogramming of adult pancreatic exocrine cells to beta-cells.Nature 455; 627-632

CHAPTER 7: HIGH BLOOD POTASSIUM

Amerine MA Ough CS 1972 Recent advances in enology. CRC Critical Reviews in Food Technology V2 issue 4407-4526.

Bellevue R Dosik H Spergel G Gussof BD1975 Pseudohyperkalemia and extreme leukocytosis. Journal of Lab.Clin. Med. 85; 660-664.

Bihari B 1995 Efficacy of low dose Naltrexone as an immune stabilizing agent for treatment of HIV/AIDS [letter] AIDS Patient Care 9; 3.

Black, R. M. (1996). Rose and Black's clinical problems in nephrology. Boston: Little, Brown, & Co.

Brown J Bourke GJ Gearty CF Finnegan A Hill M Hefferman-Fox FC Fitzgerald DE Kennedy J Childers RWBishop WJE Trulson MF Latham MC Gronin S McCann WB Clancy RE Gore I Stoudt HW Hegsted DM Stare FJ 1970 Nutritional and epidemiological factors related to heart disease. World Rev. Nutr. Diet 32.

D'Amico G Gentile MG Fellin G Manna G Cofano F1994 Effect of dietary protein restriction on the progression of renal failure: A prospective randomized trial. Nephrology Dialysis Transplantation 11; 1590-1954.

De Pronzo 1977 Impaired renal tubular potassium secretion in systemic lupus erythmatosus. Ann. Internal Medicine 86; 268-271.

Donadio JV. 2001The emerging role of omega-3 polyunsaturated fatty acids in the management of patients with IgA nephropathy. J Ren Nutr. 11(3):122-128.

Epstein FH 1960 Calcium and the kidney. Journal of Chronic Diseases 11; 255-277.

Flink EB 1983 Nutritional aspects of potassium metabolism p37-44. in;

Whang R Aikawa JK eds. Potassium its Biologic Significance. CRC Press, Boca Ratyon, Fla.

Folis RH 1942 Myocardial necrosis in rats on a potassium low diet prevented by thiamine deficiency. Bull. Johns-Hopkins Hospital. 71; 235-241.

Fored C M et al 2001 New England Journal of Medicine 345:1801-1808.

Furuya R, Kumagai H, Sakao T, Maruyama Y, Hishida A. 2002 Potassium-lowering effect of mineralocorticoid therapy in patients undergoing hemodialysis. Nephron. 92(3):576-81.

Gherardi RK 2003 Lessons from macrophagic myofasciitis: towards definition of a vaccine adjuvant-related syndrome [Article in French]. Journal: Rev Neurol (Paris) 159(2):162-4.

Giebisch G 1979 Membrane Transport in Biology. p215-298 Giebisch G editor. Springer Verlag, Berlin, NY.

HallJR Swaine RL 1972 Trends in the carbonated beverage industry. Critical Reviews in Food Technology, V2, issue 4; 517-536.

Hunter M et al 1985 Regulation of single potassium ion channels from apical membrane of rabbit collecting tubule. American Journal of Physiology – Renal Physiology 251; F725-731.

Ichinohe T Kuwahara T Yata K Seo T Suyama K Onaka H Ono T Ueda S Matsuo T 1991. Recurrent hyperkalemia in the course of rheumatoid arthritis—a case report Nippon Jinzo Gakkai Shi. Aug;33(8):811-6.

Ifudu O Markell MS Friedman FA 1992 Unrecognized pseudohyperkalemia as a cause of elevated potassium in patients with renal disease. American Journal of Nephrology 12; 102-104.

Jing SB et al 1997 Effect of chitosan on renal function in patients with chronic renal failure. Journal of Pharm. & Pharmacology 49; 721-723.

Kaufman CE Popper S 1983 Hyperkalemia. in; Whang R Aikawa JK eds. Potassium its Biologic Significance. CRC Press, Boca Raton Fl.

Knochel JP 1977 Role of glucoregulatory hormones in potassium homeostasis. Kidney International 11; 443-452.

Lasky T, Sun W, Kadry A, Hoffman MK. 2004 Mean total arsenic concentrations in chicken 1989-2000 and estimated exposures for consumers of chicken. Environ Health Perspect. 112(1):18-21.

Massola Shimizu MH, Coimbra TM, et al, 2005 N-acetylcysteine attenuates the progression of chronic renal failure, Kidney Int., 68(5): 2208-17..

Mawson AR 1985 Are rheumatoid arthritis and systemic lupus erythmatosis inversely related diseases? Medical Hypotheses 18; 377-386.

McDonald JT Margen S 1979 Wine vs ethanol in human nutrition. Fluid sodium and potassium balance. American journal of Clinical Nutrition 32; 817-822.

Moore RJ Hall CB Carlson EC Lukaski HC Klevay LM 1989 Acute renal failure and fluid retention and kidney damage in copper-deficient rats offered a high NaCl diet. Journal Lab. Clin Med. 113; 516-524.

Perneger TV, Whelton PK, Klag MJ. 1994 Risk of kidney failure associated with the use of acetaminophen, aspirin, and nonsteroidal antiinflammatory drugs. New England Journal of Medicie 331(25):1675-9.

Peterson CG 1972 Perspectives in Surgery. Lea & Febiger, Philadelphia.

Peterson L & Wright FS 1977 Effect of sodium intake on renal potassium excretion. American Journal of Physiology 233; 225-234.

Sager RH Spargo B 1955 The effects of low phosphorus ration on calcium metabolism in the rat with production of calcium citrate stones. Metabolism 4; 519.

Scribner BH & Burnell JM 1956 Metabolism 5; 468-479.

Tannen RL 1977 Relationship of renal ammonia production and potassium homostasis. Kidney International 11; 453-465.

Thompson, J., & Henrich, W. (1991). Nephrotoxic agents and their effects. In H. G. Jacobsen, G. Striker, & S. Klahr, The principles and practice of nephrology, (pp. 563 - 569). Philadelphia: B.C. Decker.

Winegrad AT Reynold AE 1958 Effects of insulin on the metabolism of glucose, pyruvate, and acetate. Journal of Biol. Chem. 233; 267.

World Health Organization 2001 Health Effects. Evaluation of certain food additives and contaminents.WHO Technical Report Series. 55th Report of the Joint FAO/WHO Expert Committee on Food Additives. p63-66.

CHAPTER 8: POTASSIUM SUPPLEMENTS

Anonymous 1994 Potassium and sodium pumps in the skeletal muscle. Laeger-Ugeskr 156; 4007-4010, 4013.

Arnett TR 2008 Extracellular pH regulates bone cell function. Journal of Nutrition 138; 4155-4185.

Baker DR et al 1964 small bowel ulceration apparently associated with thiazide and potassium therapy. Journal of the American Medical Association 190; 586-590.

Block BP Thomas MB 1978 A method for testing intestinal irritancy of sustained release potassium chloride preparations in animals. Journal Pharm. Pharmacol. 30 Suppl.70P.

Boegshold M Kotchen TA 1991 Importance of dietary chloride for salt sensitivity of blood pressure. Hypertension 17 (auppl) I 158-I161.

Carpenter CCJ, et al 1964 Green coconut water; a readily available source of potassium for the cholera patient. Bull. Cal. Sch. Trop. Med. 12; 20-21.

Chang HY, Hu YW, Yue, CSJ, Wen, YW Yeh WT, Hsu LS 2006 Effect of potassium-enriched salt on cardiovascular mortality and medical expenses of elderly men, l, American Journal of Clinical Nutrition 83(6): 1289-96.

Classen HG Marquardt P Spath M Schumacher KA Grabling B 1978 Experimental studies on the intestinal uptake of organic and inorganic magnesium and potassium compounds given alone or simultaneously. Arzneimittelforschung 28; 807-811.

Coburn JW et al 1966 Potassium depletion in heat stroke: a possible etiological factor. Milit. Med. 131; 679.

Conn HO 1970 Cirrhosis and diabetes: effect of potassium chloride administration on glucose and insulin metabolism. American Journal Med. Sci. 259; 394-404.

Dawson KG 1984 Endocrine physiologyof electrolyte metabolism. Drugs 28; suppl.1; 98.

DeLand EC Villamil MF, Maloney Jr JV. 1979 A theoretical and experimental study of ionic shifts induced by K depletion and replacement. Journal of Theoretical Biology 76; 31-51.

Dluhy RG Axelrod L Underwood RH Williams GH 1972 Studies of the control of plasma aldosterone concentration in normal man. J. Clin. Invest. 51; 1950-1957.

Dow, Steven W., DVM, et al 1992 Taurine Depletion and Cardiovascular Disease in Cats Fed a Potassium-Depleted, Acidified Diet, l, American Journal of Veterinary Research, 53(3):402-405.

Ellis D Banner B, Janosky JE Feig PU 1992 Potassium supplementation attenuates experimental hypertensive renal injury. Journal of the American Society of Nephrology 2; 1529-1537.

Ellison HS Holley HL 1953 Hypokalemia due to insufficient dietary intake. Am. Practicioner 4; 6-8.

Fabry P et al 1968 Meal frequency and ischemic heart disease. Lancet 2; 190.

Frassetto LA Morris C Sebastian A 1997 Potassium bicarbonate reduces urinary nitrogen excretion in postmenopausal women. Journal of Clinical Endocinology and Metabolism 82; 254-259.

Frassetto LA Nash E Morris RC Sebastian A 2000 Comparative effects of potassium chloride and bicarbonate on thiazide-induced reduction in urinary calcium excretion. Kidney International 58; 748-752.

Friedberg CK Diseases of the Heart, 3rd edition. WB Saunders, Philadelphia.

Gennari J 1998 Hypokalemia (a review). Current Concepts 339; 451-458.

Giebisch G 1979 Membrane Transport in Biology. p215-298 Giebisch G editor. Springer Verlag, Berlin, NY.

Golf SW, et al. 1998 On the Significance of Magnesium in Extreme Physical Stress, Cardiovasc Drugs Ther, 12;197-202.

Green, DM, Ropper AH, Kronmal RA, Psaty BM, Burke GL 2002 for The Cardiovascular Health Study. Serum potassium level and dietary potassium intake as risk factors for stroke. Neurology. 59: 314-320.

Griffith RS et al 1987 Success of L-lysine therapy in frequently recurring herpes simplex infection. Dermatologica 175; 180-183.

Hamill-Ruth RJ & McGary R 1996 Magnesium repletion and its effect on potassium homeostasis in critically ill adults: results of a double-blind, randomized, controlled trial. Critical Care Medicine. 24; 38-45.

Houston MC 2002 The Role of Vascular Biology, Nutrition and Nutraceuticals in the Prevention and Treatment of Hypertension. JANA, 1(Suppl): 5-71.

Jehle S Zanetti A Muser J Hulter HN Krapf R 2006 Partial neutralization of the acidogenic Western diet with potassium citrate increases bone mass in postmenopausal women with osteopenia. Journal of the American Society of Nutrition. 17; 3213-3222.

Jansson, B 1990 Dietary, Total Body and Intracellular Potassium-To-Sodium Ratios and Their Influence on Cancer. Cancer Detection and Prevention 14(5); 563-565.

Kohvakka A Luurila O Gordin A Sundberg S 1989 Magnesium. Magnesium 8; 71-76.

Labow BI Wiley W Souba MD 2000 Glutamine. World Journal of Surgery 24; 1503-1513.

Lane HW et al 1978 Effect of physical activity on human potassium metabolism in a hot and humid environment. American Journal of Clinical Nutrition 31; 838-843.

Lin SH, Chiu JS, Hsu CW, Chau T. 2003 A simple and rapid approach to hypokalemic paralysis. American Journal of Emergency Medicine. 21(6):487-91.

Luft FC Zemel MB Sowers JA Fineberg NS Weinberger MH 1990 Sodium bicarbonate and sodium chloride: effects on blood pressure and electrolyte homeostasis in normal and hypertensive man. Journal of Hypertension 8; 663-670.

MacIntyre I Davidson D 1958 The production of secondary potassium depletion, sodium retention, nephrocalcinosis and hypercalcemia by magnesium deficit. Biochem. Journal 70; 456-462.

Manitius A 1965 Some physiological effects of magnesium deficiency p28. in: Electrolytes and Cardiovascular Diseases, Bajusz E, editor. S. Karger, New York.

Masters RD Coplan M 1998 Water Treatment with Silicofluorides and enhanced lead uptake, Fluoride, 31, No 3, Aug. or NeuroToxicology 21 (6); 1091-1100.

McCarty MF 2004 Should we restrict chloride rather than sodium? Medical Hypotheses 63;138-148.

Morgan TO 1979 Potassium replacement: Supplements or potassium sparing diuretics? Drugs 18; 218-215.

Morris RC et al 1999; Differring effects of supplemental KCl and KHCO3: pathophysiological and clinical implications. Seminars in Nephrology 19; 487-493.

Mosely DS Osborne B 2003 Ingestion of potassium chloride crystals causes hyperkalemia and hemorrhajic gastritis. Emergency Medicine News 25; 18-20.

Muhlbauer RC Li F 1999 Effect of vegetables on bone metabolism. Nature 401; 343-344.

Norris W, Kunzelman KS, Bussell S, Rohweder L, Cochran RP. 2004 Potassium supplementation, diet vs pills: a randomized trial in postoperative cardiac surgery patients. Chest. Feb;125(2): 404-409.

Palva IP et al 1972 Drug induced malabsorbtion of vitamin B12. Malabsorbtion and deficiency of B12 during treatment with slow-release potassium chloride. Acta. Med. Scand. 191, 355-357.

Penry JT Manore MM 2008 Choline: an important micronutrient for maximal endurance exercise performance? Sport Nutrition-Exercise Metabolism. 18; 191-203.

Petersen VP 1963 Potassium and magnesium turnover in magnesium deficiency. Acta Med. Scand. 174; 595-604.

Ring K Grimm E Schwartz M 1976 Interrelationship between transport of L-aspartate and potassium ions into the cell (author's translation, article in German). Arzneimmittelforsch. 26; 1195-1201.

Rogers, Sherry 1992 Chemical sensitivity: breaking the paralyzing paradigm: how knowledge of chemical sensitivity enhances the treatment of chronic disease. Internal Medicine World Report, 7(8):13-41.

Romanski SA, McMahon MM. 1999 Metabolic acidosis and thiamine deficiency. Mayo Clin Proc. 74(3): 259-63.

Rude RK1998 Magnesium deficiency: A cause of heterogenous disease in humans, Journal of Bone and Mineral Research, 13(4): 749-758.

Sebastian, A. et al. 1994 Improved mineral balance and skeletal metabolism in postmenopausal women treated with potassium bicarbonate. The New England Journal of Medicine. 330: 1776-1781.

Schlebusch, H., et al, 1992 Bioavailability of magnesium as magnesium-orotate and magnesium-hydroxycarbonate", Med Welt, 43; 523-8.

Schwartz J Weiss S 1990 Dietary factors and their relation to respiratory symptoms. American Journal of Epidemiology 132; 67-76.

Selye H, et al 1945 Experimental nephrosclerosis, prevention with ammonium chloride. Lancet 1; 301H304.

Selye H Bajusz E 1958 Provocation and prevention of potassium deficiency by various ions. Proceedings of the Soc. Exptl. Biol. and Med. 98; 580-583.

Smith SR Klotman PE Svetley LP 1992 Potassium chloride lowers blood pressure and causes natriuresis in older patients with hypertension. Journal of the American Society of Nephrology. 2; 1302-1309.

Soler NG et al 1972 Potassium balance during treatment of diabetic ketoacidosis. Lancet 300 isue #7779, 665-667.

Stamler, Jeremiah and Cirillo, Massimo 1997 Dietary Salt and Renal Stone Disease, The Lancet 349 :506-507.

Stedwell RE Allen KM Binder LS 1992 Hypokalemic paralyses: a review of the etiologies, pathophysiology, presentation, and therapy. Am J Emerg Med, 10(2):143-148.

Sukenik S Neumann L Buskila D Kleiner-Baumgarten A Zimlichman S Horowitz J 1990 Dead sea bath salts or the treatment of rheumatoid arthritis. Clinical Exp. Rheumatology 8; 353-357 (from the abstract).

Takacs BE 1998 ,Potassium: A New Treatment for Premenstrual Syndrome. Journal of Orthomolecular Medicine. 13(4): 215-222.

Tannen RL 1977 Relationship of renal ammonia production and potassium homostasis. Kidney International 11; 453-465.

Tekol Y 2006 Is systemic hypertension only a sign of chronic sodium chloride intoxication? Medical Hypotheses 67; 630-638.

Varner JA, et al 1998 Chronic administration of aluminum-fluoride or sodium fluoride to rats in drinking water: Alterations in neuronal and cerebrovascular integrity. Brain Research 784 (1-2); 284_298.

Walsh CR Larson MG Leip EP VasanRS Levy D 2002 Blood potassium and heart serum potassium and risk of cardiovascular disease. Archives of Internal Medicine. 162; 1007-1012.

Welfare W Sasi P English M 2002 Challenges in managing profound hypokalemia. BMJ 2002;324:; 269-270.

White RJ 1970 Potassium supplements on the exchangeable potassium in chronic heart disease. British Medical Journal 3; 141-142.

Williams CL Meck WH Heyer DD Loy R 1998 Hypertrophy of basal forebrain neurons and enhanced visuospatial memory in perinatally choline supplemented rats. Brain Research 794: 225-238,.

Williams MH 1999 Facts and fallacies of purported ergogenic amino acid supplements. Clin. Sports Med. 18(3); 633-649.

Zeisel SH -Heng Mar M Juliette C. Howe JC Holden JM 2003 Concentrations of Choline-Containing Compounds and Betaine in Common Foods. The American Society for Nutritional Sciences J. Nutr. 133: 1302-1307.

CHAPTER 9: HORMONAL REGULATION OF POTASSIUM AND SODIUM

Abbrecht PH 1972 Cardiovascular effects of chronic potassium deficiency in the dog. American Journal of Physiology 223; 555-560.

Abernethy JD 1979 Sodium and potassium in high blood pressure. Food. Technology. 33; 57-59.

Aguilera G. Lightman, S.L. Kiss, A 1993 Regulation of the Hypothalamic-Pituitary-Adrenal Axis During Water Deprivation. Endocrinology 132; 241.

Ahluwalia J Tinker A Clapp LH Duclien MR Abromav AY Pope S Nobles M Segal AW 2004 The large conductance Ca-activated K channel is essential for immunity. Nature 427; 853-858.

Bartlett GR MacKay EM 1949 Insulin stimulation of glycogen formation in rat abdominal muscle. Proceedings. Society Experimental. Biology Med. 71; 493-495.

Bauer JH Gauntner WC 1974 Effect of potassium chloride on plasma renin activity and plasma aldosterone during sodium restriction in normal man. Kidney International 15; Kidney Int. 15; 286.

Relman AS Schwartz WB 1952 The Effect of DOCA on Electrolyte Balance in Normal Man and Its Relation to sodium Chloride Intake. Yale Journal of Biological Medicine 24; 540.

Bennett CM et al 1968 Micropuncture study of nephron function in the rhesus monkey. Journal of Clinical Investigation 47; 203.

Biglieri EG Lopez JM 1977 Adrenocorticotropin and plasma aldosterone concentration and deoxycorticosterone in man. Ann. New York Academy of Science 297; 361-372.

Bonner G Autenreith R Mari-Grez M Rascher W Gross F 1981 Hormone. Research. 14; 87.

Braley LM Williams GH 1977 Rat adrenal cell sensitivity to angiotensin II, ACTH alpha 1-24, and potassium. American Journal of Physiology Endo. 233; E402.

Brown RD Strott CA Liddle GW 1972 Site of stimulation of aldosterone biosynthesis by angiotensin and potassium. Journal of Clinical Investgation 51; 1413-1418.

Clark WS et al 1956 The relationshp of alterations in mineral and nitrogen metabolism to disease activity in a patient with rheumatoid arthritis. Acta Rheum. Scand. 2; 193-212.

Cope CL Llaurado JG 1954 The occurence of electrocortin in human urine. British Medical. Journal 1; 1290.

Cox RH 1977 Carotid artery mechanics and composition in renal and DOCA hypertension in the rat. Cardiovascular Medicine 2; 761-768.

Dale SL Melby JC 1974 Altered adrenal steroid genesis in "low renin" essential hypertension. Transactions of the Association of American Physicians 87; 248-257.

Damasco MC Diaz F Anal JP Lantos CP 1979 Acute effects of three natural corticosteroids on the acid-base and electrolyte composition of urine in adrenalectomized rats. Acta Physiol. Latin Am. 29; 305

Desaulles P 1958 Comparison of the effects of aldosterone, cortexone and cortisol on adrenalectomized rats under various salt loads. in; International Symposium on Aldosterone (Muller AF & O'Conner, eds.) pp 29-38. Little Brown Co., Boston.

Dluhy RG Axelrod L Underwood RH Williams GH 1972 Journal of Clinical Investigation 51; 1950.

Dolman D, Edmonds CJ. 1975 The effect of aldosterone and the renin-angiotensin system on sodium, potassium and chloride transport by proximal and distal rat colon in vivo. Journal of Physiology 250(3): 597-611.

Donowitz M Binder, HJ 1976 Effect of Enterotoxins of Vibrio Cholerae, Escherichia coli, & Shigella Dienteriae Type 1 on Fluid and Electrolyte Transport in Colon. Journal of Infectious Diseases 134; 135.

Douglas J Mansen J Catt KJ 1978 Relationships between plasma renin activity and plasma aldosterone in the rat after dietary electrolyte changes. Endocrinology 103; 60.

Ellinghaus K 1971 Sodium and potassium balance during the administration of desoxycorticosterone in dogs with differing intakes. Pfluegers Arch. 322; 347-354.

Elman, R., et al. 1952 Intracellular and Extracellular Potassium Deficits in Surgical. Patients. Ann. Surgery 136; 111.

Eppinger A 1939 Z. Arzneimittelforschung 36; 672, 709,

Fang J Madhaven S Cohen H Alderman H 2000 Serum potassium and cardiovascular mortality. Journal of Gen. Int. Medicine 15; 885-890.

Farrell G 1958 Regulation of aldosterone secretion. Phys. Rev. 38; 709.

Flatman JA Clausen T 1979 Combied effects of adrenaline and insulin on active electrogenic Na+ and K= transport in rat soleus muscle. Nature 281 ; 580-581.

Folis RM et al 1942 The production of cardiac and renal lesions in rats by a diet extremely deficient in potassium. American Journal of Pathology 18; 29.

Fraser R 1971 Effect of steroids on the transport of electrolytes. Biochem. Society Symposium 32; 101-1212.

Fraser R Lantos CP 1978 18-hydroxycorticosterone: a review. J. Steroid Biochem. 9; 273-286

Fuller PJ Pressley L Adam WF Funder JW 1976 16, 18-dihydroxydeoxycorticosterone and the binding of aldosterone to mineralocorticoid receptors in kidney of adrenalectomized rats. Journal Steroid Biochemistry 7: 387-390.

Gadsby DC 2004 Spot the difference. Nature 427; 795-797.

Gann DS Cruz JF Casper AGT Bartter FC 1962 Mechanism by which potassium increases aldosterone secretion in the dog. American Journal Phys. 202; 991.

Gann DS Mills IH Bartter 1960 On the hemodynamic parameter mediating increase in aldosterone secretion in the dog. Fed. Proceedings 19; 605-610.

Glaz E & Vecsei P 1971 Aldosterone, Pergamon Press, NY.

Gornall AC et al 1960 The influence of estrogen and progesterone on urinary sodium and aldosterone excretion. Acta Endocrin. 35 Suppl. 51; 157.

Grekin RJ Terris JM Bohr DF 1980 Electrolyte and hormonal effects of deoxycorticosterone acetate in young pigs. Hypertension 2; 326-332.

Grim CE, Luft FC, Miller JZ, Meneely GR, Battarbee HD, Hames CG, Dahl LK 1980 Racial differences in blood pressure in Evans County, Georgia: relationship to sodium and potassium intake and plasma renin activity. J Chronic Dis. 33(2):87-94.

Helman SI I'Neil BG 1977 transport characteristics of renal collecting tubules:- Influence of DOCA and diet. American Journal of Physiology 293; F544-558.

Hiatt N et al 1972 The effect of potassium chloride infusion on insulin secretion in vivo. Hormone Metabolism Research 4; 64.

Hornyck A Meyer P Milliez P 1973 Angiotensin, vasopressin, and cyclic AMP: affects on sodium and water fluxes in rat colon. American Journal of Physiology 224: 1223.

Jiang Y Lee A Chen J Gadene M Chait T MacKinnon R 2002 Crystal structure and mechanism of a calcium-gated potassium channel Nature 417; 515-522.

Kernan RP 1980 Cell Potassium. John Wiley & Sons, NY.

Knochel JP 1977 Role of glucoregulatory hormones in potassium homeostasis. Kidney International 11; 443..

Lans HS et al 1952 The relation of serum potassium to erythrocyte potassium in normal subjects and patients with potassium deficiency. American Journal Med. Sci. 223; 65-74.

LaCelle PL Morgan ES Atwater EC 1964 Arthritis Rheum. 7; 321.

Lamson E et al 1956 Aldosterone excretion of normal, schizophrenic and psychoneurotic subjects. Journal of Clinical Endocr. Metab. 16; 954.

Libretti A 1965 in; Electrolytes and Cardiovascular Diseases (Bajusz E, ed.) Vol. 1, Williams and Wilkins, Baltimore, pp. 121-134.

Linas SL Peterson LN Anderson RJ Aisenbrey GA Simon FR Berl T 1979 Mechanism of renal potassium conservation in the rat. Kidney International 15; 601-611.

Majima, M I Hayashi T Fujita H Ito S Nakajima 1999 Kallikrein-kinin system prevents the development of hypertension by inhibiting sodium retention. Immunopharmacology 44 issue 1+2; 145-152.

Matsuoka Y et al 1981 Studies of death in autopsied cases with rheumatoid arthritis. from; New Horizons in Rheumatoid Arthritis (Shiokawa Y Abe T & Yamauchi Y, eds.) Exerpta Medica International Cong. Series #535.

May CN Lewis PS Horth CE 1979 Radioimmunoessay of plasma 18-hydroxy-11-deoxycorticosterone and its response to ACTH. Clin. Endocrinol. 11; 399-412.

Melby JC et al 1971 18 hydroxy-deoxycorticosterone in human hypertension. Circ. Res. 18; Suppl. II, 143.

Melby JC et al 1972 18-hydroxy 11 deoxycorticosterone (18 OH-DOC) secretion in experimental and human hypertension. Recent Progress in Hormone Resarch. 28; 287-351.

Melby JC Dale SL 1976 New mineralocorticoids and adrenocorticoids in hypertension. American Journal of Cardiology 38; 805-813.

Melby JC Dale SL. 1977 Role of 18-hydroxy-11-deoxycorticosterone and 16 alpha, 18-dihydroxy-11-deoxycorticosterone in hypertension. Mayo. Clin. Proc. May;52(5):317-22.

Merrill DC Skelton MM Cowley AW,Jr. 1986 Humoral control of water and electrolyte excretion during water restriction. Kidney International 29; 1152-1161.

Messerli PT Wojciech N Masanobu H Genest J Boucher R Kuchel O Rojoortega JM 1977 Effects of angiotensin II on steroid metabolism and hepatic blood flow in man. Circulation Research 40; 204-207.

Mikosha AS Pushkarov IS Chelnakova IS Remennikov GYA 1991 Potassium Aided Regulation of Hormone Biosynthesis in Adrenals of Guinea Pigs Under Action of Dihydropyridines: Possible Mechanisms of Changes in Steroidogenesis Induced by 1,4, Dihydropyridines in Dispersed Adrenocorticytes. Fiziol. [Kiev] 37; 60.

Miller C 2001 See potassium run. Nature 414; 23-24.

Moore TJ Braley LM Williams GH 1978 Stimulation of 18-hydroxy-11-deoxycorticosterone secretion by angiotensin II and potassium. Endocrinology 103; 152-155.

Muller J 1979 11beta hydroxylation of 18 – hydroxy – 11 – deoxycorticosterone by rat adrenal tissue: zone specificity and effect of sodium snd potassium restriction. Journal of Steroid Biochemistry 13; 253-257.

Nichols MG Fraser R Hay G Mason P Torsney B 1966 Urine electrolyte response to 18-hydroxy-11-deoxycorticosterone in normal man. Clinical Science Mol. Med. 53; 493-498.

Nichols MG Fraser R Hay G Mason P Torsney B 1977 Urine electrolyte response to 18-hydroxy-11-deoxycorticosterone in normal man. Clin. Sci. Mol. Med. 53(5); 493-498.

Noskov SY Berneche S Roux B 2004 Control of ion selectivity in potassium channels by electrostatic and dynamic properties of cabonyl ligands. Nature 431; 830-834.

Oddie CJ et al 1972 Plasma deoxycorticosterone levels in man with simultaneous measurement of aldosterone corticosterone, cortisol and eoxyotisol. Journal of Clinical Endocrinol. Metab. 34; 1039-54

Oliver WJ Cohen EL Neel JV 1975 Blood pressure, sodium intake, and sodium related hormones in the Yanomamo indian's "no salt culture". Circulation 52; 146-151.

O'Neil RG & Helmans SI 1977 Transport characteristics of renal collecting tubules: influence of DOCA and diet. American Journal of Physiology 233; 544-558.

Parker CR Jr. et al 1980 Hormone production during pregnancy in the primigravid patient. American Journal of Obstet. Gynecol. 58; 26-30.

Parker CR Jr. et al 1981 Plasma concentrations of 11-deoxycorticosterone in women during menstrual cycle. Obstet. Gynecol 58; 26-30.

Pearce JW et al 1969 Evidence for a humoral factor modifying the renal response to blood volume expansion in the rat. Can. Journal of Physiological Pharm. 47; 377-386.

Peterson CG 1972 Perspectives in Surgery Lea & Febiger, Philadelphia.

Peterson L & Wright FS 1977 Effect of sodium intake on renal potassium excretion. American Journal of Physiology 233; 225-234.

Pospisilova J 1970 Influence of mineralocorticoids on collagen synthesis in subcutaneous granuloma in adrenalectomized and non-adrenalectomized mice. Physiol. Bohemoslov. 19; 539-543.

Potts WTW Perry G 1964 Osmotic and Ionic Regulation in Animals. MacMillan, NY.

Pratt JH 1982 Angiotensin II in potassium mediated stimulation of aldosterone secretion in the dog. Journal of Clinical. Investigation. 70; 667

Rastmanesh R 2008 A pilot study of potassium supplementation in treatment of hypokalemic patients with rheumatoid arthritis: a randomized, double-blinded, placebo controlled trial. The Journal of Pain 9; 722.

Rubini ME Chojnocki RF 1972 J. Clin. Nutr. 25; 96.

Ruch TC Fulton JF 1960 Medical Physiology and Biophysics. W.B. Saunders and Co., Phijl & London.

Schacht RG et al 1971 Renal mechanism for DOCA escape in man BulL. N.ew York Academy of Medicine 47; 1233.

Schambelan M Biglieri EC 1972 Deoxycorticosterone production and regulation in man. Journal of Clinical Endocrinology and Metabolism 34; 695-703.

Schneider EG Radke KJ Ulderich DA Taylor RE 1985 Effect of osmolality on aldosterone secretion. Endocrinology 116; 1621-1626.

Scribner BH Burnell JM 1956 Metabolism 5; 468-479.

Selye H Sylvester O Hall CE Leblond CP 1944 J. Am. Med. Assoc 124; 201.

Sharp GUG Leaf A 1966 in; Recent Progress in Hormone Research.(Pincus G, ed.) Academic Press, NY.

Shi N Ye S Alain A Chen L Jiang Y 2006 Atomic structure of a Na+- and K+ - conducting channel. Nature 440; 570-574.

Solomon AK 1962 Pumps in the living cell. Scientific American 207; 100-108.

Sparano F et al 1978 18-hydroxy-11-deoxycorticosterone response to insulin in normal man. Journal of Steroid Biochemistry 9; 1061-1063.

Squires RD Huth EJ 1959 Journal of Clinical. Investigation. 38; 1134.

Stanbury SW Gowenlock AH Mahler RF 1958 Aldosterone (Muller AF O'Connor CM eds) pp 155-166 Little Brown & Co, Boston

Tan, S.Y.; Mulrow, P.J. 1978 Regulation of 18 Hydroxydeoxy- Corticosterone in the Rat."Endocrinology 102: 1113,.

Venning EH Dyrenfurthen JC Beck J 1957 Effect of anxiety upon aldosterone excretion in man. J.Clinical Endocrinology and Metabolism. 17; 10.

Wambach G Higgins JR 1979 Effect of progesterone on serum and tissue electrolyte concentration in DOCA-treated rats. Hormone Metabolism Research 11; 258-259.

Weber CE 1974 Potassium in the etiology of rheumatoid arthritis and heart infarction. Journal Applied Nutrition. 26; 41.

Weber CE 1998 Cortisol's purpose Medical Hypotheses 51; 289-292.

Wehling M, Armanini D, Strasser T, Weber PC. 1987 Effect of aldosterone on sodium and potassium concentrations in human mononuclear leukocytes. Am J Physiol. 1987 Apr;252(4 Pt 1):E505-508.

Williams GH Braley LM Underwood RH 1976 The regulation of plasma 18 hydroxy 11-deoxycorticosterone in man. Journal of Clinical Investigation 58; 221-231.

Williams GH Dluhy RG 1972 American Journal of Medicine. 53; 595.

World Health Organization 1960 Epidemiological and Vital Statistics Report. WHO 13.

Wright FS 1977 Sites and mechanisms of potassium transport along the renal tubule. Kidney International 11; 415-432.

Zhou et al 2001 Chemistry of ion coordination and complex at 2.0 angstrom resolution. Nature 414; 43-48.

CHAPTER 10: POTASSIUM PHYSOLOGY

Abbrecht PH Vander AJ 1970 Effects of chronic potassium deficiency on plasma renin activity. Journal of Clinical Investigation 49; 1510-1516.

Abbrecht PH 1972 Cardiovascular effects of chronic potassium deficiency in the dog. American Journal of Physiology 223; 555-560.

American Medical Association 1951 Handbook of Nutrition, 2nd Ed. Blakiston Co., NY.

Amlal H Wang Z Soleimani M 1998 Potassium depletion down regulates chloride - absorbing transporters in rat kidney. Journal of Clinical Investigation 101; 1045-1054.

Baumann K & Muller J !972 Effect of potassium intake on the final steps of aldosterone biosynthesis in the rat. Acta Endocrinol. 69; 701 & 718.

Bellevue R Dosik H Spergel G Gussof BD 1975 Pseudohyperkalemia and extreme leukocytosis, Journal of Lab.Clin. Med. 85; 660-664.

Brown MR et al 1944 Muscular paralysis and electrocardiographic abnormalities resulting from potassium loss in chronic nephritis. Journal of the American Medical association 124; 545.

Cannon PR et al 1951 Influence of potassium on tissue protein synthesis. Metabolism 1; 49-57.

Cockel R, Kendall MJ, Becker JF, Hawkins CF: 1971 Serum biochemical values in rheumatoid disease. Ann Rheum Dis 30(2):166-70.

Cope CL 1964 Adrenal Steroids and Disease. JB Lippincott Co., Philadelphia.

Davis WH 1970 Does potassium deficiency hold a clue to metabolic disorders associated with liability to heart disease?. South African Med. Journal 44; 1297.

de Witte TJ Geerdink PJ Lames CB Boerbooms AM van der Korst JK 1979 Hypochlorhydria and hypergastrinaemia in rheumatoid arthritis. Annals of the Rheumatic Diseases 38, 14-17.

Eckel RE et al 1954 Lysine as a muscle cation in potassium deficiency. Arch. Biochem. Biophys. 52; 293.

Epstein FH 1960 Calcium and the kidney. Journal of Chronic Diseases 11; 255-277.

Evans BM et al 1957 Alkalosis in sodium and potassium depletion. Clinical Science 16; 53.

Folis RM et al 1942 The production of cardiac and renal lesions in rats by a diet extremely deficient in potassium. American Journal of Pathology 18; 29.

Folis RH, Jr. 1953 The pathology of potassium deficiency. 73; 241.

Frassetto L Morris RC Jr. Sellmeyer DE Todd K Sebastan 2001 Diet, evolution and aging The pathophysiologic effects of the post-agricultural inversion of the potassium-to-sodium and base-to-chloride ratios in the human diet. Europian Journal of Nutition 40 (no. 5); 200-213.

Galvez OG; Bay WH; Roberts BW; Ferris TF 1977. The hemodynamic effects of potassium deficiency in the dog. Circ. Res. 40. I-11 – I-16.

Gann DS et al 1964 Control of aldosterone secretion by change of body potassium in normal man. American Journal of Physiology 207; 104.

Gardner LI et al 1950 The effect of potassium deficiency on carbohydrate metabolism. Journal Lab & Clin. Med. 35; 592-602.

Gardner LI MacLachlan EA Berman H 1952 Effect of potassium deficiency on carbon dioxide, cation, and phosphate content of muscle. Journal of General Physiology 36; 153-159.

Gardner LI 1953 Experimental potassium depletion. Journal Lancet 73; 190.

Garella S et al 1970 Saline - resistant metabolic alkalosis or chloride - wasting nephropathy. Ann. Internal Medicine 73; 31-38.

Hartung EF Steinbrocker O 1935 Gastric acidity in chronic arthritis Ann. Intern. Med. 9; 252-257.

Heaney RP 2006 Role of Dietary Sodium in Osteoporosis. Journal of the American College of Nutrition 25, No. 90003, 271S-276S.

Holman RL et al 1960 Arterioscelerosis - the lesion. American Journal of Clinical Nutrition 8; 85-94.

Iacobellis M et al 1956 Free amino acid patterns of certain tissues from potassium and/or protein - deficient rats. Amer. Journal Physiology 185 ; 275.

Ifudu O Markell MS Friedman EA 1992 Unrecognized pseudohyperkalemia as a cause of elevated potassium in patients with renal disease. American Journal of Nephrology 12; 102-104.

Jasani BM & Edmond CJ 1971 Kinetics of potassium distribution in men using isotope dilution and whole body counting. Metabolism 20; 1099-1106.

Kark RM 1958 Some aspects of nutrition and the kidney. American Journal of Nutrition 25; 698-707

Kotchen TA Guthrie GP Jr. Galla JH Luke RG Welch WJ 1983 Effects of NaCl on renin and aldosterone responses to potassium depletion. American Journal of Physiology 244 (2); E164-169.

Labow BI Soula WW 2000 World Journal of Surgery 24; 1503.

Lambie AT 1964 Renal mechanisms of potassium depletion. Proceedings Nutr. Soc. 24; 63-73

Luke RG Wright FS Fowler N Kashgarian M & Giebisch GH 1978 Effect of potassium depletion on renal tubular chloride transport in the rat. Kidney International 14; 414-427.

Marcus DF et al 1968 A comparative study of various hyperglycemic agents in potassium deficient rats. Proceedings of the Society Experimental Biol. Med. 127; 533-538.

Molnar Z et al 1962 Cardiac changes in the potassium depleted rat. Arch. Pathol. 74; 339-347.

Naslund PH & Hultin T 1971 Structural and functional defects in mammalian ribosomes after potassium deficiency. Biochem. Biophys. Acta 254; 104.

Nickel JF et al 1953 Renal function during sodium deprivation. Journal of Clinical Investigation 32; 68-79.

Noergaard A Kjeldsen K Clausen T 1981 Potassium depletion decreases the number of 3H-oubain binding sites and active Na-K transport in skeletal muscle. Nature 293; 739-741.

Ono I Hukuoka T Onodera I 1964 The effects of varying dietary potassium on the electrocardiogram and blood electrolytes in young dogs. Jap. Heart Journal 5; 272.

Patrick J & Bradford b 1971 A comparison of leucocyte potassium content with other measurements in potassium - depleted rabbits. Clinical Science 42; 415-421.

Rector FC Jr. et al 1955 The mechanism of ammonia excretion during ammonium chloride acidosis. Journal of Clinical Investigation 34; 20.

Rhodin JAG 1971 Structure of the kidney. in; Diseases of the Kidney (Strauss MB & Welt LG, editors) Little Brown & Co., Boston.

Rinehart KE et al 1968 Effect of dietary deficiency of potassium on protein synthesis in the young chick. Journal of Nutrition 95; 627-632.

Rowinski P 1960 Potassium in the animal organism - Proceedings of the 6th Congress of the International Potash Institute, Amsterdam, p381-433.

Rubini ME 1961 Water excretion in potassium - deficient man. Journal of Clinical Investigation 40; 2215-2224.

Rubini ME Chojnacki RE 1972 Principles of parenteral therapy. American. Clinical . Nutrition 25; 96-113.

Rusk HA Weichselbaum TE 1939 Changes in serum potassium in certain allergic states. JAMA 112, No. 23; 2395-2398.

Rowe JW et al 1980 Effect of experimental potassium deficiency on glucose and insulin metabolism. Metabolism 29; 448-502.

Scribner BH Burnell JM 1956 Metabolism 5; 468-479.

Sealey JE et al 1970 Potassium balance and the control of renin secretion. Journal of Clinical Investigation 49; 2119-2127.

Smith SG Lasater TE 1950 Diabetes insipidus like condition produced in dogs with potassium deficient diet. Proc. Soc. Exptl. Biol. Med. 74; 427-431.

Southon S Heaton FW 1981 Changes in cellular and subcellular composition during potassium deficiency. Comparative Biochemistry and Physiology 72a; 415-419.

Spergel et al 1967 Potassium on the impaired glucose tolerance in chronic uremia metabolism. Metabol. Clin. Ex. 16; 581-585

Surawicz B 1968 The role of potassium in cardiovascular therapy. Medical. Clinics North America. 52; 1103-1113.

Strauss MB Welt LG, editors 1971 Diseases of the Kidney, Vol II, Little Brown & Co., Boston.

Syrjanen S, Lappalainen R, Markkanen H 1986 Salivary and serum levels of electrolytes and immunomarkers in edentulous healthy subjects and in those with rheumatoid arthritis. Clin Rheumatol. 5(1):49-55.

Tannen RL 1977 Relationships of renal ammonia production and potassium homeostasis. Kidney International 11; 453-465.

Tate CL Bagdon WJ Bokelman DVM 1978 Morphological abnormalities in potassium - deficient dogs. American Journal Pathology 93; 103-116.

Truong L et al 1973 Influence of dietary protein on skeletal muscle growth of normal and potassium - chloride depleted young rats. Nutr. Reports Int. 7; 655-664.

Weber CE 2005 Eliminate infection (abscess in teeth with cashew nuts. Medical Hypotheses 65; 1200.

Welt LG et al 1958 The prediction of muscle potassium from blood electrolytes in potassium depleted rats. Tr. A. Am Physicians 71; 750.

Welt LG et al 1960 Consequences of potassium depletion. Journal of Chronic Dis. 11; 213-254.

Wohl MG Goodhart RS 1968 Modern Nutrition in Health and Disease, 4th edition. Lea & Febiger

Zhu K Devine A Prince RL 2004 The effects of high potassium consumption on bone mineral density in a prospective cohort study of elderly postmenopausal women. Osteoporosis International 20 (no. 2); 336-340.

Zusman RM Keiser HR 1980 Regulation of prostaglandin E2 synthesis by angiotensin II, potassium, osmolality, and dexamethasone. Kidney International 17; 277-283.

CHAPTER 11: HISTORY OF RHEUMATOID ARTHRITIS RESEARCH

Ahluwalia J et al 2004 The large conductance Ca-activated K channel is essential for immunity. Nature 427: 853-858.

Balandraud N Meynard JB Sooran H Mugnier B Reviron D Reviron D Roudier J Roudier Chantal 2003 Epstein Barr virus load in the peripheral blood of patients with rheumatoid arthritis. Arthritis and Rheumatism 48; 1223-1228

Bihari B 1995 Efficacy of low dose Naltrexone as an immune stabilizing agent for treatment of HIV/AIDS [letter] AIDS Patient Care 9; 3.

Bjarnason I, Peters TJ. 1996 Influence of anti-rheumatic drugs on gut permeability and on the gut associated lymphoid tissue. Baillieres Clin Rheumatol 10(1):165-76.

Campbell IK O'Donnell K Lawlor KE Wicks IP 2001 Severe inflammatory arthritis and lymphadenoppathy in the absence of TNF. Journal of Clinical Investigation 107; 1519-1527.

Casanova JL Abel L 2002 Annu. Rev. Immunol. 20; 581.

Childers NF 1981 Childer's Diet to Stop Arthritis. Horticultural Publications, Somerset Press, Inc., Somerville, New Jersey.

Cobb S 1962 Hostility and its control in rheumatoid diseases. Arth. & Rheum 5; 290.

Cole, AA Chubinskaya, S Luchene, LJ Chlebek, K Orth, MW Greenwald, RA Kuettner, KE Schmid TM 1994 Doxycycline disrupts chondrocyte differentiation and inhibits cartilage matrix degradation.(39 references and summary) Arthritis and Rheumatism 37: 12: 1727-1734.

Cordain L. Toohey L. Smith MJ. Hickey MS. 2000 Modulation of immune function by dietary lectins in rheumatoid arthritis. [Review] [114 refs] Source British Journal of Nutrition. 83(3): 207-17.

Das UN 2000 Newer uses of glucose-insulin-potassium regime. Med Sci. Monit. 6; 1053-1055.

Dessein PH Joffe BI Stanwicx AE Moomel Z 2001 Hyposecretion of the adrenal androgen dehydroepiandrosterone sulfate and its relation to chemical variables in inflammatory arthritis.Arthritis Research 3; 183-187.

Diehl HW 1994 Cetyl myristoleate isolated from Swiss albino mice: an apparent protective agent against adjuvant arthritis in rats. J. Pharm.Sci. 83(3):296-9.

Dong CH Banks J 1975 New Hope for the Arthritic. Ballantine Books, New York.

Donta ST et al 2004 Benefits and harms of doxycycline treatment for Gulf War veterans' illnesses A randomized, double-blind, placebo-controlled trial. Annals of Internal Medicine 141; 85-94.

Lee S-J Yeo W-H Yun B-S Yoo I-D 1998 (date of first online publication) Isolation and sequence analysis of new peptoboi boietusin, from Boletus spp. Journal of Peptide Science 5; 374-378.

Espinosa-Morales R, Escalante A 1998 Diagnostic confusion caused by hepatitis C: hemochromatosis presenting as rheumatoid arthritis. J Rheumatolology ;25(12):2459-63.

Eyring H Dougherty TF 1957 Molecular Mechanisms in Inflammation and

Stress -"Science in Progress" 10 series p181-194, Yale University Press, New Haven, Conn.

Forman R. 1981 Medical resistance to innovation. Medical Hypotheses. 7:1009-17.

Gardner LI MacLachlan EA Berman H 1952 Effect of potassium deficiency on carbon dioxide, cation, and phosphate content of muscle. Journal of General Physiology 36; 153-159.

Gerard HC Branigan PJ Schumacher HR Jr. Hudson AP 1998 A synovial Chlamydia trachomatis in patients with reactive arthritis/Reiter's syndrome are viable but show aberrant gene expression. Journal of Rheumatology. 25; 734-742.

Go CHU Clarke T-A Cunha BA 2000 Persistent septic arthritis with recurrent bacteremia as a result of a tolerant strain of Staphylococcus aureus. Heart and Lung 29; 383-385.

Gompel LL Smith AA Charles PJ Rogers W Soon-Shiang J Mitchell A Dore C Taylor PW Mackworth-Young CG 2006 Single-blind randomized trial of combination antibiotic therapy in rheumatoid arthritis. The Journal of Rheumatology 33; 224-227.

Gorman JD 2006 Smoking and rheumatoid arthritis: another reason to just say no. Arthritis Rheum. 54; 10-13.

Jick SS Lieberman ES Rahman MU Choi HK 2006 Glucocorticoid use, other associated factors, and the risk of tuberculosis. Arthritis and Rheumatism (arthritis Case and Researtch) 55; 19-26.

Kahn A, Jr. 1965 potassium deficiency and chronic pyelonephritis. Journal of the . Arkansas Medical Society 61; 341 342.

Kloppenburg, M Mattie, H Douwes, N Dijkmans, BAC Breedveld. FC 1995 Minocycline in the treatment of rheumatoid arthritis: Relationship of serum concentrations to efficacy. Journal of Rheumatology 22: 4: 611-616.

Liu PT Stenger S Li H Wenzel L Tan BH Krutzik SR Ochoa MT Schauber J Wu K Meinken C Kamen DL Wagner M Bals R Steinmeyer Zugel U Gallo RL Eisenberg D Hewison M Hollis BW Adams JS Bloom BR Modlin RL 2006 Toll-like receptor triggering of a vitamin D-mediated human antimicrobial response. Science 311; 1770-1773.

Louro MO, Cocho JA, Mera A, Tutor JC. 2000 Immunochemical and enzymatic study of ceruloplasmin in rheumatoid arthritis. J Trace Elem Med Biol. 14(3):174-8.

Marshall TG Marshall FE 2004 Sarcoidosis succumbs to antibiotics – implications for autoimmune disease. Autoimmunity Reviews 4; No.4; 295-300.

McCord JM 1974 Free radicals and inflammation: protection of synovial fluid by superoxide dismutase. Science 185; 529.

Mikkelsen WM,Chairman 1981 Arthritis and Rheumatism 24; 159, 133-134.

Mikosha, AS Pushkarov IS.Chelnakova IS Remennikov GYA 1991 Potassium Aided Regulation of Hormone Biosynthesis in Adrenals of Guinea Pigs Under Action of Dihydropyridines: Possible Mechanisms of Changes in Steroidogenesis Induced by 1,4, Dihydropyridines in Dispersed Adrenocorticytes. Fiziol. [Kiev] 37: 60.

Millman M 1972 An allergic concept of the etiology of rheumatoid arthritis. Ann. Allerg. 30; 135-140.

Nalbandian RM et al 1981 Polymyalgia rheumatica and giant cell arteritis-Rational diagnosis and treatment predicated on disordered prostaglandin metabolism. Medical Hypotheses 7; 1169-1182,

Nicolson, GL. Nasralla, MY, De Meirleir K, Gan, R., Haier J 2003 Evidence for Bacterial and Viral Co-Infections in Chronic Fatigue Syndrome Patients. Journal of Chronic Fatigue Syndrome 2003; 11(2):7-20.

Olakanmi O Britigan BE Schlesinger LS 2000 Gallium disrupts iron metabolism of mycobacteria residing within human macrophages. Infect. Immun. 68; 5619-5627.

Permin H. et al 1981 Possible role of histamine in rheumatoid arthritis. Allergy 36; 435-436.

Phillips PE 1975 Virologic studies in rheumatoid arthritis. Rheumatology vol. 6.

Poehlmann KM 2002 Rheumatoid Arthritis: the Infection Connection. Satori Press, 904 Silver Spur Road #323, Rolling Hills Estates, CA 90274.

Ramírez AS Rosas A Hernández-Beriain JA Orengo JC Saavedra P de la Fe C Fernández A Poveda JB 2005 Relationship between rheumatoid arthritis and Mycoplasma pneumoniae: a case–control study. Rheumatology 44(7):912-914.

Randolph TG 1976 Clinical Ecology (Dickey LD ed.) p201-212. CC Thomas, Springfield.

Rashid T Ebringer A 2008 Rheumatoid arthritis in smokers could be linked to Proteus urinary tract infections. Medical Hypotheses 70; 975-980.

Rastmanesh R 2008 A pilot study of potassium supplementation in treatment of hypokalemic patients with rheumatoid arthritis: a randomized, double-blinded, placebo controlled trial. The Journal of Pain 9; 722-731.

Sacerdote P Manfredi B Gaspani L Panerai AE 2000 The opioid antagonist naloxone induces a shift from type 2 to type 1 cytokine pattern in BALB/cJ mice. Blood. 95(6): 2031-2036.

Schaeverbeke, T Clerc, M Lequen, L Charron, A Bebear, C Debarbeyrac, B Bannwarth, B Dehais, J Bebear. C 1998 Genotypic characterization of seven strains of Mycoplasma fermentans isolated from synovial fluids of patients with arthritis. Journal of Clinical Microbiology 36: 5, :1226-1231.

Schmidt JE 1959 Medical Discoveries, Who and When. Charles CT Thomas, Springfield Il.

Schuschke DA, Saari JT, West CA, Miller FN 1994 Dietary copper deficiency increases the mast cell population of the rat. Proc Soc Exp Biol Med. Dec;207(3): 274-7.

Selye H et al 1944 Hormonal production of arthritis. Journal of the American Medical Association 124; 201.

Selye H 1949 Further studies concerning the participation of the adrenal cortex in the pathogenesis of arthritis. British Medical Journal 2; 1129.

Seong S Choi C Woo J Bae K Joung C Uhm W Kim T Jun J Yoo D Lee J Bae S 2007 Incidence of Tuberculosis in Korean Patients with Rheumatoid Arthritis (RA): Effects of RA Itself and of Tumor Necrosis Factor Blockers. J Rheumatology 2007;34:706–711.

Siegel, LB Gall. EP 1996 Viral infection as a cause of arthritis. American Family Physician 54: 6 :2009-2015.

Sinaii N, Cleary SD, Ballweg ML, Nieman LK, Stratton P Crohn's 2002 RA may be from coeliac from gluten disease which may be more common than thought Journal: Human Reproduction 17(10):2715-2724.

Singh SB Davis AS[1] Taylor GA Vojo Deretic V 2006 **Human** IRGM induces autophagy to eliminate intracellular mycobacteria. Science 313; 1438-1441.

Sorenson JRJ 1980 Copper chelates as possible active metabolites of the antiarthritic and antiepiletic drugs. Journal of Applied Nutrition 32; 4-25.

Staub RH Pongratz G Scholmerick J Kees F Schaible TF Antoni C Kalden JR Lorenz H-M 2003 Long term anti tumor necrosis factor antibody therapy in rheumatoid arthritis patients sensitizes the pituitary gland and favors adrenal androgen secretion. Arthritis and Rheumatism 48; 1504-1512.

Turnbull JA 1944 Study of 127 cases of arthritis. American Journal of Digestive Disease 11; 122-130.

Turner CD 1955 General Endocrinology, 2nd edition. WB Saunders Co. Philadelphia.

Wallingford WR McCarty DJ 1971 Differential membranolytic effects of microcrystalline sodium urate and calcium pyrophosphate dihydrate. The Journal of Experimental Medicine, 133, 100-112.

Weber CE 2005 Eliminate infection (abscess) in teeth with cashew nuts. Medical Hypothesis 65; 1200.

Weismann G 1972 Lysosomal mechanisms of tissue injury in arthritis. New England Journal of Medicine 286; 141.

Welt LG et al 1960 Consequences of potassium depletion. Journal of Chronic Disease 11; 213-254.

Wilson C Ebringer Aahmidi K et al 1995 Shared amino acid sequences beween major histocompatibility complex class II glycoproteins , type XI collagen, andProteus mirabolis in rheumatoid arthritis. Ann. Rheum. Dis. 54; 216-220.

Woods JW Welt LG Hollander W Jr. 1961 Susceptibility of rats to experimental pyelonephritis during potassium depletion. Journal of Clinical Investigation 40; 599-602.

Wyburn-Mason R 1979 The naeglerial (free living amoebic) causation of rheumatoid disease and many human cancers. A new concept in medicine. Medical Hypothesis 5; 1237-1249.

Zeller M 1949 Rheumatoid Arthritis; Food Allergy as a Factor. Ann. Allerg. 7; 200-205.

Zoli A, Altomonte L, Caricchio R, Galossi A, Mirone L, Ruffini MP, Magaro M. 1998 Serum zinc and copper in active rheumatoid arthritis: correlation with interleukin 1 beta and tumour necrosis factor alpha. Clin Rheumatology17(5): 378-82.

Zussman BM 1966 Food hypersensitivity simulating rheumatoid arthritis. South Med. J. 59; 935-939.

CHAPTER 12: THE FUNCTION OF CORTISOL

Adler, S. 1970 An Extrarenal Action of Aldosterone on Mammalian Skeletal Muscle. American Journal of Physiology 218: 616.

Aguilera, G.; Lightman, S.L.; Kiss, A. 1993 Regulation of the Hypothalamic-Pituitary-Adrenal Axis During Water Deprivation. Endocrinology 132: 241.

Barger, A.C.; Berlin, R.D.; Tulenko, J.F. 1958 Infusion of aldosterone, 9 alpha fluorohydrocortisone, and antidiuretic hormone into the renal artery of normal and adrenalectomized unanesthetized dogs: Effect on electrolyte and water excretion. Endocrine. 62: 804.

Barseghian, G.; Levine, R 1980 Effect of corticosterone on insulin and glucagon secretion by the isolated perfused rat pancreas.Endocrinology 106: 547.

Barseghian, G.; Rachmiel, L.; Epps, P 1982 Direct effect of cortisol and cortisone on insulin and glucagon secretion. Endocrinology 111: 1648.

Bauman K Muller J 1972 Effect of potassium on the final status of aldosterone biosynthesis in the rat. I 18-hydroxylation and 18hydroxy dehydrogenation. II beta-hydroxylation. Acta Endocrin. Copenh. 69; I 701-717, II 718-730.

Beilin B Shavit Y Razumovsky J Wolloch Y Zeidel A Bessler H. 1998 Effects of Mild Perioperative Hypothermia on Cellular Immune Responses. Anesthesiology 89(5); 1133-1140.

Bell J Moore GJ. 1974 Effects of High Ambient Temperature on Various Stages of Rabies Virus Infection in Mice. Infect. Immun. 10(3); 510–515.

Beutler, B.; Cerami, A 1987 Cachectic: more than a tumor necrosis factor. New Engl. Journal of Medicine 316: 379.

Beutler, B. Cerami, C 1987 The Endogenous Mediator of Endotoxin Shock. Clin. Res. 35: 192.

Bihari B 1995 Efficacy of low dose Naltrexone as an immune stabilizing agent for treatment of HIV/AIDS. [letter]. AIDS Patient Care 9; 3.

Besedovsky, H.O.; Del Rey, A.; Sorkin, E 1984 Integration of activated immune cell products in immune endocrine feedback circuits. p. 200 in Leukocytes and Host Defense Vol. 5 [Oppenheim, J.J.; Jacobs, D.M., eds]. Alan R. Liss, New York.

Besedovsky, H. del Ray A; Sorkin E Dinerello CA1986 Immunoregulatory feedback between interleukin-1 and glucocorticoid hormones.Science 233: 652.

Bartlett, GR MacKay EM 1949 Insulin stimulation of glycogen formation in rate abdominal muscle. Proc. Exp. Biological Medicine 71: 493.

Boykin J de Torrent A Erickson A Robertson G Schrier RW 1978 Role of plasma vasopressin in impaired water excretion of glucocorticoid deficiency. Journal of Clinical Investigation 62: 738.

Chambers JW Georg RH Bass AD 1965 Effect of hydrocortisone and insulin on uptake of alpha aminoisobutyric acid by isolated perfused rat liver. Mol. Pharmacol. 1: 66.

Charnes AN Donowitz MJ 1976 Prevention and reversal of cholera enterotoxin-induced intestinal secretion by methylprednisolone induction of Na-K-ATPase. Journal of Clinical Invest. 57: 1590.

Civen M Leeb RM Wishnow RM Morin RJ 1980 Effects of dietary ascorbic acid and vitamin E deficiency on rat adrenal cholesterol ester metabolism and vitamin E deficiency on rat adrenal cholesterol ester metabolism and corticosteroidogenesis. Int. Journal of Vitamin Nutr. Res. 50: 70.

Clark IA Virilizier JL Carswell EA Wood PR 1981 Possible importance of macrophage-derived mediator in acute malaria. Aus. Infect. Immun. 32: 1058.

Colwell RR 1996 Global climate and the infectious disease: the cholera paradigm. Science 274; 2125-2031.

Curry DL Bennett LL 1973. Dynamics of insulin release by perfused rate pancreas effects of hypophysectomy, growth hormone, adrenocorticotropic hormone and hydrocortisone. Endocrinology 93: 602.

Curtis MJ Flack IM Harvey SI 1980 The effect of escherichia coli endotoxin on the concentration of corticosterone and growth hormone in the plasma of the domestic low. Res. Vet. Sci. 28: 123.

Da Prato RA Rothschild J 1986 The AIDs virus as an opportunistic organism inducing a state of chronic relative cortisol excess: Therapeutic implications. Med. Hypotheses. 21: 253.

Damasco MC Diaz F Anal JP Lantos CP 1979 Acute effects of three natural corticosteroids on the acid base and electrolyte composition of urine in adrenalectomized rats. Acta. Physiol. Latino Am. 29: 305.

Davies E Keyon CJ Fraser R 1985 The role of calcium ions in the mechanism of ACTH stimulation of cortisol synthesis. Steroids 45: 557.

De Pasquale A Coste G Trovat A 1979 Effect of prostaglandins on the increased corticosterone output induced by caffeine in the rat. Prostaglandins Med. 3: 97.

Deronzo R 1983 The effect of dexamethasone on renal potassium excretion and acute potassium tolerance. Endocrinology 113: 1690.

Devoe IW 1980 The interaction of polymorphonuclear leukocytes and endotoxin in meningococcal disease: A short review. Canadian Journal of Microbiol. 26: 729.

Dingman JF Gonzalez-Auvert Ahmed ABJ Akinura A 1965 Antidiuretic hormone in adrenal insufficiency. Journal of Clinical Investigation 44: 1041.

Dollman D Edmonds CJ 1975 The effect of aldosterone on chloride transport by proximal and distal rat volon in vivo. Journal of Physiology. London, 250: 597.

Donowitz M Binder HJ 1976 Effect of enterotoxins of vibrio cholerae, Escherichia coli, & Shigella dienteriae type 1 on fluid and electrolyte transport in colon. Journal of Infectious Diseases. 134: 135.

Doyle MP, Campylobacter in Foods. In Campylobacter Infection in Man and Animals. CRC, Boca Raton.

Dvorak M 1971 Plasma 17-hydroxycorticosteroid levels in healthy and diarrheic calves. British Veterinarian Journal 127: 372.

Evans GW 1973 Copper homeostasis in the mammalian system. Physiol. Review 53: 535.

Fairchild SL Shannon K Kwan E Mishell RI 1984 T Cells derived gucocorticosteroid lymphocytes and a T-cell hybridoma. Journal of Immunology 132: 821.

Field M Fromm D Wallace DK Greenough WB, III 1969 Stimulation of active chloride secretion in small intestine by cholera exotoxin. Journal of Clinical Invest. 48: 24a.

Field T et al 2005 Cortisol decreases and serotonin and dopamine increase following massage therapy. International Journal of Neuroscience. 115; 1397-1413.

Finklestein, R.A 1973 Cholera. CRC Critical Reviews in Microbiology 2: 553.

Finlay GJ Boothe RJ Marbrook J 1979 Antibody responses of human lymphocytes in vitro; Enhancing effects of hydrocortisone. Austr. Journal of Exp. Biol. Med. 57: 597.

Flohe L Beckman R Giertz H Loschen G Oxygen Centered Free Radicals as Mediators of Inflammation. p. 405, in Oxidative Stress (Sies H, ed) Academic Press, NY.

Gardner LI 1953 Experimental potassium depletion. Journal of Lancet 73: 190.

Govan CD Jr. Darrow DC 1946 The use of potassium chloride in the treatment of diarrhea in infants. Journal of Pediatrics 38: 541.

Ghosh S Chatterjee GC 1979 Superoxide dismutase activity in Vibrio cholerae eltor in relation to oxygen toxicity and bactericidal action of nitrofurantoin. Journal of General Appl. Microbiology 25: 367.

Glass AI 2006 New hope for defeating retrovirus. Scientific American 294; 46-55.

Goodrun KJ Berry LJ 1978 The effect of glucocorticoid antagonizing factor on hepatoma cells. Pro. Soc. Exp. Biol. Med. 159: 369.

Gorbman A Dickhoff WW Vigna SR Clark NB Muller AF Comparative Endocrinology. John Wiley and Sons, New York.

Gregoriadis G Sourkes TL 1970 Regulation of hepatic copper in the rat by the adrenal gland. Canadian Journal of Biochem. 48: 160.

Gutenbrunner C Schreiber U 1987 Circadian variations of urine excretion and adrenocortical function in different states of hydration in man. Prog Clin Biol Res. ;227A:309-16.

Hall NR Goldstein AL 1984 Endocrine regulation of host immunity. p. 536, in; Immune Modulation Agents and Their Mechanisms, (eds Fenichel, RL and Chirigos, MA) Marcel Dekker, NY.

Hanson DE Murphy PA Silicano R Shin HS. 1983 The effect of temperature on the activation of thymocytes by interleukin I & II. Journal of Immunol. 130; 216,

Hirahata, F. The Role of Lipocortins in Cellular Function as a Second Message of Glucocorticoids, in Antiinflammatory Steroid Action, Schleseimer, R.P.; Claman, H.N.; Oronsky, A.L., eds. Academic Press, San Diego, NY.

Hornyck, A.; Meyer, P.; Milliez, P. 1973 Angiotensin, vasopressin, and cyclic AMP: Effects on sodium and water fluxes in rat colon. American Journal of Physiology. 224: 1223,

Houck, J.C.; Sharma, V.K.; Patel, Y.M.; Gladner, J.A 1968 Induction of collagenolytic and proteolytic activities by antiInflammatory drugs in the skin and fibroblasts. Biochemical Pharmacology 17: 2081.

Husband AJ Brandon MR Dascelles AK1973 The effect of corticosteroid on absorption and endogenous production of immunoglobulins in calves. Aust. Journal of Exp. Biol. Med. Sci. 55: 707.

Jirapongsananuruk O Melamed I Leung DY 2000 Additive immunosuppressive effects of 1,25-dihydroxyvitamin D3 and corticosteroids on TH1, but not TH2, responses. J Allergy Clin Immunol. 106(5): 981-5.

Johnson KJ Ward PA 1972 The requirements for serum complement in the detoxification of bacterial endotoxin. Journal of Immunol. 108: 611.

Jones RS Howell EV Eik-Nesk 1959 Inactivation by plasma of ACTH releasing property of C-14 labeled bacterial polysaccharide. Proc. Soc. of Exper. Biol. Med. 100: 328.

Kernan, RP 1980 Cell Potassium. John Wiley, New York.

Kinney FT Kull FJ 1963 Hydrocortisone stimulated synthesis of nuclear RNA in enzyme induction. Proc. Nat. Aad. Sci. U.S. 50: 493.

Kjeldson-Kragh J Hangen M Borchgrevink CF Laerum E Eek M Mowinkel P Hovi K Forre O 1991 Controlled trail of fasting and one year vegetarian diet in rheumatoid arthritis. Lancet 338: 899.

Kluger MJ. 1978 The evolution and adabtive value of fever. American Sci. 66; 38-43.

Knight RP, Jr. Kornfield DS Glaser GH Bondy PK 1955 Effects of intravenous hydrocortisone on electrolytes in serum and urine in man. Journal of Clinical Endocrinology 15: 176,

Knochel JP 1977 Role of glucoregulatory hormones in potassium homeostasis. Kidney International 11: 443.

Kokshchuk GI Pakhmurnyi BA 1979. Role of glucocorticoids in regulation of the acid-excreting function of the kidneys. Fiziol. Z H SSR I.M.I.M. Sechenova 65: 751,

Lukaseqycz OA Prohaska JR 1983 Lymphocytes from copper deficient mice exhibit decreased mitogen reactivity. Nutrition Research 3: 335,.

Luke RG Wright FS Fowler N Kashgarian M Giebisch GH 1978 Effects of potassium depletion on renal tubular chloride transport in the rat. Kidney Int. 14: 414-427.

Mach RS Fabre J 1955 Clinical and metabolic effects of aldosterone. p. 736 in CIBA Foundation Colloquia on Endocrinology, VIII, 16: 361,.

Manchester KL Sites of hormonal regulation of protein metabolism. p. 229, Mammalian Protein [Munro, H.N., Ed.]. Academic Press, New York.

Mannel DJ 1982 Possible role of endotoxin in mediating host resistance. Klin. Wochenschr. 60: 752.

Mason PA Fraser R Morton JJ 1977 The effect of sodium deprivation and of angiotensin II infusion on the peripheral plasma concentration of 18Hydroxy-corticosterone, aldosterone, and other corticosteroids in man. Steroid Biochemistry 8: 799.

Mekalanos JJ Swartz DJ Pearson GDN Hartford N Groyne F Wilde M 1983 Cholera Toxin Genes: Nucleotide sequence, deletion analysis and vaccine development. Nature 306: 551.

Melby JC Egdahl RH Spink WW 1960 Secretion and metabolism of cortisol after injection of endotoxin. Journal of Lab. Clinical Medicine. 56: 50.

Mendelsohn FA Mackie C 1975 Relation of intracellular K+ and steroidogenesis in isolated adrenal zona glomerulosa and fasciculata cells. Clinical Sci. Mol. Medical 49: 13.

Meng J Wyss AR Dawson MR Zhai R 1994 Primitive fossil rodent from inner Mongolia and its implications. Nature 370; 134-136.

Michie HR Spriggs DR Monogue KR Sherman ML Revhang A O'Dwyer ST Arthur K Dinerello CA Cerami A Wolff SM Kufe DW Wilmore DW 1988 Surgery 104: 280.

Mikosha AS Pushkarov IS Chelnakova IS Remennikov GYA 1991 Potassium aided regulation of hormone biosynthesis in adrenals of guinea pigs under action of dihydropyridines: Possible mechanisms of changes in steroidogenesis induced by 1,4, dihydropyridines in dispersed adrenocorticytes. Fiziol. [Kiev] 37: 60.

Milenkovic L Rettori V Snyder GD Beutler B McCann SM 1989 Cachectic alters anterior pituitary hormone release by a direct action in vitro. Proc. Nat. Acad. Sci. 86: 2418.

Mishel RI Bradley LM Chen YU Grabstein GH Shiigi SM 1979 Glucocorticosteroid Response Modifying Factors Derived form Accessory Cells. Annals NY Acad Sci. 332; 433.

Moore RN Goodrum KJ Couch R Berry LJ 1978 Factors affecting macrophage function: glucocorticoids antagonizing factor. J. Reticuloendothel Soc. 23; 321.

Moore, R.N.; Shackleford, G.M.; Berry, L.J. 1985 Glucocorticoid Antagonizing Factor. Handbook of Endotoxin vol. 3, Cellular Biology of Endotoxin p. 123, Berry L.J., ed. Elsevier, Amsterdam,

Mora, R· Makoto Iwata Bertus Eksteen, Si-Young Song, Tobias Junt, Balimkiz Senman, Kevin L. Otipoby, Aya Yokota Hajime Takeuchi, Paola Ricciardi-Castagnoli, Klaus Rajewsky, David H. Adams, Ulrich H. von Andrian 2006 Generation of Gut-Homing IgA-Secreting B Cells by Intestinal Dendritic Cells. Science 314; 1157 – 1160.

Muller AF Oconnor CM, ed. 1958 An International Symposium on Aldosterone, page 58. Little Brown & Co.

Newby TJ Stokes CR Local Immune Response of the Gut., CRC, Boca Raton.

Newsholme EA Leech AR, Biochemistry for the Medical Sciences. John Wiley & Sons, New York.

Nishida, S.; Matsumuru, S.; Horino, M.; Ogama, H.; Tenku, A 1977 The variations of Plasma corticosterone/cortisol ratios following ACTH stimulation or dexamethasone administration in normal men. Journal of Clinical Endocrinol. Metab. 45: 585.

Oelkers W Boelke T Bahr V Exner P Faust B Harendt H1988 Dose response relationships between plasma adrenocorticotropin (ACTH), cortisol, aldosterone, and 18hydroxy-corticosterone after injection of ACTH or human corticotropin-releasing factor in man. Journal of Clinical Endocrinology & Metabolism 66: 181.

Onsrud M Thorsby E 1981 Influence of in vivo hydrocortisone on some blood lymphocyte subpopulations 1. effect on natural killer cell activity. Scand. J. Immunol. 13; 573-579.

Oyama, T.K.; Toyooka, Y.; Sato, S.; Kondo 1978 "Effect of endotoxic shock on renal and hormonal functions. Can.Anaesth. Soc. Journal 25: 380.

Palacios R Sugawara I1982 Hydrocortisone Abrogates proliferation of T-Cells in autologous mixed lymphocyte reaction by rendering the interleukin-2 producer cells unresponsive to interleukin-1 and unable to synthesize the T-Cell growth factor. Scandinavian Journal of Immunology 15: 25.

Pierce NF Sacci JB, Jr. Alving CR Richardson EC 1986 Rev. Infect. Disease 6:563.

Piletz JE Herschman HR1983 Hepatic metallothionein synthesis in neonatal ottled-brindled mice.Biochem. Genet. 21: 465.

Plotsky PM Sapolsky Otto S 1986 Inhibition of immunoreactive corticotropin-releasing factor secretion into the hypophysial portal circulation by delayed glucocorticoid feedback. Endocrinology 119: 1126.

Portanova R1972 Release of ACTH from Isolated Pituitary Cells: An energy dependant process. Proc. Soc. Exp. Biol. Med. 140: 825.

Posey WC Nelson HS Branch B Pearlman DS 1978 The effects of acute corticosteroid therapy for asthma on serum immunoglobulin levels. J. Allergy Clin. Immunol. 62: 340.

Pospisilova J Pospisil M 1970 Influence of mineralocorticoids on collagen synthesis in subcutaneous granuloma in adrenalectomized and nonadrenalectomized mice. Physiologia Bohemoslovaca 19: 539.

Quigley ME Yen SSC 1979 A mid-ay surge in cortisol concomitant with food intake in women. Journal of Clinical Endocrinol. Metab. 49: 945.

Rastmanesh R 2008 A pilot study of potassium supplementation in treatment of hypokalemic patients with rheumatoid arthritis: a randomized, double-blinded, placebo controlled trial. The Journal of Pain 9; 722.

Reiser S Ferretti RJ Fields M Smith JC 1983 Roles of dietary fructose in the enhancement of mortality and biochemical changes associated with copper deficiency in rats. American Journal of Clinical Nutrition 38; 214.

Relman, A.S; Schwartz, W.B 1952 The effect of DOCA on electrolyte balance in normal man and Its relation to sodium chloride Intake. Yale Journal of Biological Medicine 24:540.

Sandle GI Keir MG Record CO 1981 The effect of hydrocortisone on the ttransport of water, sodium, and glucose in the jejunum. Scandinavian Journal of Gastroenterol. 16: 667.

Schlaghecke R Kornely E Wollenhaupt J Specker C 1992 Glucocorticoid receptors in rheumatoid arthritis. Arthritis Rheum 35: 740.

Schneider EG Radke KJ Ulderich DA Taylor RE, Jr. 1985 Effect of osmolality on aldosterone secretion. Endocrinology 116: 1621.

Scholer D Birkhauser M Pyetremann A Riondel AM Vallotton MB Muller AF 1973 Response of plasma aldosterone to angiotensin II, ACTH, and potassium in man. Act. Endocrinol. 72: 293.

Small PM Täuber MG Hackbarth CJ Sande MA. 1986 Influence of body temperature on bacterial growth rates in experimental pneumococcal meningitis in rabbits. Infection and Immunity 52; 484-487.

Smith NC1989 The role of free oxygen radical in the expulsion of primary infections of Nippostrongylus brasiliensis. Parisitology Research 75: 423.

Soffer LJ. Dorfman RI Gabrilove JL. The Human Adrenal Gland., Febiger, Phil.

Starch BC Hill CH 1965 Hormonal induction of ceruloplasmin in chicken serum. Comparative Biochem. Physiol. 15: 429.

Stith RD McCalum RE 1986 General effect of endotoxin on glucocorticoid receptors in mammalian tissues. Circ. Shock 18; 301-309.

Tai Y Decker RA Marnane WG Charney AN 1981 Effects of methylprednisolone on electrolyte transport by rat ileum in vitro. American Journal of Physiology 240-G346: 70.

Tan SY Mulrow PJ 1978 Regulation of 18 hydroxydeoxy-corticosterone in the rat. Endocrinology 102: 1113.

Tobian L, Jr. Binion JT 1954 Artery wall electrolytes in renal and DCA hypertension. Journal of Clinical Investigation 23: 1407.

Torpy DJ Ho JT 2007 Corticosteroid-binding globulin gene polymorphisms: clinical implications and links to idiopathic chronic fatigue disorders. Clinical Endocrinology 67; 161–167.

Ueda Y Honda M Tsuchiya M Watanabe H Izumi Y Shiratsuchi T Inoue T Hatano M 1982 Response of plasma ACTH and adrenocortical hormones to potassium loading in essential hypertension. Jpn Circ J. 46(4): 317-22.

Uehara A Gottschall PE Dahl RE Akira A 1987 Interleukin 1 stimulates ACTH release by an indirect action which requires endogenous corticotropin releasing factor. Endocrinology 121; 1580-1582.

Weber CE 1983 Corticosteroid Regulation of Electrolytes. Journal of Theor. Biology 104: 443.

Weber, C.E 1984 Copper response to rheumatoid arthritis. Medical Hypotheses 15: 333-348.

Weber CE 2007. Creation of a local 'fever' using an infrared lamp to cure a tooth abscess. Medical Hypotheses 68(2):458. Epub 2006 Sep 26.

Welt LG Hollander W, Jr. Blythe WB 1960 Consequences of potassium depletion. Journal of Chronic Diseases 11: 213.

Wilson DL. 1957 Direct effects of adrenal corticosteroids on the electrolyte content of rabbit leucocytes. American Journal of Physiology. 190: 104,.

Yeh KY Moog F 1977 Influence of the thyroid and adrenal glands on the growth of the intestine of the suckling rat and on the development of intestinal alkaline phosphatase and disaccharidase activities.. Journal of Exp. Zoology 200: 337-349..

Zellner M Hergovics N Roth E Jilma B Spittler A Oehler R. 2002 Human monocyte stimulation by experimental whole body hyperthermia. Wien. Klin. Wochenschr. 114(3); 73-75.

Printed in the United States
By Bookmasters